Eye Emergencies

The practitioner's guide

2nd Edition

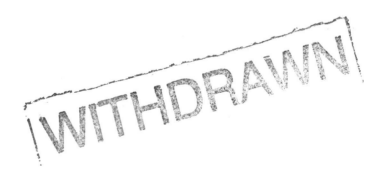

eBook version also available

Eye Emergencies: The practitioner's guide
2nd Edition
ISBN: 9781907830952

*For the full range of M&K Publishing books
please visit our website:* www.mkupdate.co.uk

Eye Emergencies

The practitioner's guide

2nd edition

Dorothy Field
Julie Tillotson
Emma Whittingham

Eye Emergencies: The practitioner's guide
2nd edition
Dorothy Field, Julie Tillotson & Emma Whittingham

ISBN: 9781905539-95-6

First published 2008, this edition published 2015

British Library Catalogue in Publication Data
A catalogue record for this book is available from the British Library.

Notice
Clinical practice and medical knowledge constantly evolve. Standard safety precautions must be followed, but, as knowledge is broadened by research, changes in practice, treatment and drug therapy may become necessary or appropriate. Readers must check the most current product information provided by the manufacturer of each drug to be administered and verify the dosages and correct administration, as well as contraindications. It is the responsibility of the practitioner, utilising the experience and knowledge of the patient, to determine dosages and the best treatment for each individual patient. Any brands mentioned in this book are as examples only and are not endorsed by the publisher. Neither the publisher nor the authors assume any liability for any injury and/or damage to persons or property arising from this publication.

Disclaimer
M&K Publishing cannot accept responsibility for the contents of any linked website or online resource. The existence of a link does not imply any endorsement or recommendation of the organisation or the information or views which may be expressed in any linked website or online resource. We cannot guarantee that these links will operate consistently and we have no control over the availability of linked pages.

To contact M&K Publishing write to:
M&K Update Ltd · The Old Bakery · St. John's Street
Keswick · Cumbria CA12 5AS

Tel: 01768 773030 · Fax: 01768 781099
publishing@mkupdate.co.uk
www.mkupdate.co.uk

Designed & typeset in 11pt Usherwood Book by Mary Blood
Printed in England by H&H Reeds, Penrith.

Contents

List of illustrations   vii

About the authors   viii

About this book   ix

Acknowledgments   x

Chapter 1: Anatomy and physiology of the eye   1
Protection of the eye *1*
The conjunctiva *4*
The lacrimal apparatus *5*
The external eye muscles *7*
The eye *8*
The optic pathways *15*
References *16*

Chapter 2: Initial assessment   17
Ophthalmic triage *17*
Recording an eye history *19*
Vision testing *20*
Basic eye examination kit *25*
Eye examination with a pen torch *26*
Slit lamp examination *31*
References *32*
Differential diagnosis guide: acute red eyes *33*
Visual Disturbance assessment chart *34*

Chapter 3: Differential diagnosis of emergency eye conditions   37
Chemical injuries *38*
Major eye injuries *44*
Acute glaucoma *48*
Ophthalmia neonatorum *53*
Orbital infections *55*
Sudden painless loss of vision *58*
Sudden loss of vision with pain *66*
Hypopyon and hyphaema *69*
References *72*

Chapter 4: Major accidents and injuries   75
Accidents and injuries *75*
Infections *88*
Recurrent erosion of the cornea *92*
Corneal inflammations *93*
Corneal infections *96*
Uveal tract disorders *101*
Visual perception disorders *104*
Post-operative related eye problems *107*
References *108*

Chapter 5: Non-urgent eye conditions   111
Face and eyelids *111*

Conjunctival problems *123*

Differential diagnosis guide: types of conjunctivitis *129*

Scleral problems *135*

Other presentations *137*

References *139*

Chapter 6: Drugs commonly used for acute eye conditions   141

General principles *141*

Pregnancy and lactation *142*

Eye drops and contact lens wear *142*

Acute glaucoma *143*

Antibiotics *144*

Antihistamine and mast cell stabilisers *145*

Antivirals *146*

Steroids *146*

Lubricants *147*

Local anaesthetics *148*

Pupil dilators *148*

Diagnostic eye drops *150*

References *151*

Chapter 7: Ophthalmic pain   153

General principles *153*

Severe aches *153*

Stabbing pain *154*

Children and eye pain *156*

Ophthalmic sensation table *150*

References *157*

Chapter 8: Concluding notes   159

The changing face of ophthalmic ED provision *159*

Telephone triage *159*

Instructions for all eye emergency patients on discharge *161*

Practitioner responsibilities *162*

Patient Assessment – Eye Accident and Emergency flow chart *163*

Signs & Symptoms based Ophthalmic Triage Tool *164*

Record of Telephone Triage Advice – Eye Unit *166*

Chapter 9: Ophthalmic procedures   167

Irrigating an eye *167*

Checking the pH of an eye *169*

Everting an eyelid *169*

Checking eye movements *171*

Checking for relative afferent pupillary defect (RAPD) *172*

Visual fields by confrontation *173*

Seidel test to detect a wound leak *174*

Corneal staining with fluorescein *175*

Application of heat to the eyelids *176*

References *178*

Glossary of ophthalmic terms   179

Index   185

List of illustrations

1.1   The eyelid *2*

1.2   Conjunctival fornices *4*

1.3   The lacrimal apparatus *5*

1.4   The tear film *6*

1.5   The external eye muscles *7*

1.6   The whole eye *8*

1.7   The cornea *9*

1.8   Drainage angle *10*

1.9   The optic pathways *15*

3.1   Severe chemical injury *39*

3.2   Penetrating injury *44*

3.3   Acute glaucoma *50*

3.4   Neovascular (rubeotic) glaucoma *52*

3.5   Preseptal cellulitis *56*

3.6   Orbital cellulitis *57*

3.7   Central retinal artery occlusion *60*

3.8   Central retinal vein occlusion *62*

3.9   Vitreous haemorrhage *64*

3.10 Hypopyon *69*

3.11 Hyphaema *70*

4.1   Full thickness eyelid laceration *78*

4.2   Corneal foreign body *85*

4.3   Herpes zoster ophthalmicus *88*

4.4   Acute dacryocystitis *90*

4.5   Corneal neovascularisation - contact lens overuse *94*

4.6   Bacterial corneal ulcer *97*

4.7   Herpes simplex keratitis (dendritic ulcer) *99*

4.8   Acanthamoeba keratitis *100*

5.1   Bell's palsy *112*

5.2   Blepharitis *115*

5.3   Stye *120*

5.4   Chalazion *121*

5.5   Viral conjunctivitis *127*

5.6   Subconjunctival haemorrhage *131*

9.1   Cardinal eye positions *172*

About the authors

Dorothy Field RGN, OND, BSc(Hons), PGCE(A), MA, EdD
Retired Lecturer Practitioner, Bournemouth Eye Unit

Julie Tillotson RGN, OND, BSc(Hons)
Independent and Supplementary Prescriber
Advanced Nurse Practitioner
Bournemouth Eye Unit and Community Eye Clinic Adam Practice

Emma Whittingham Adv Dip, BSc(Hons), MSc
Nurse Practitioner, Independent and Supplementary Prescriber
Advanced Nurse Practitioner
Bournemouth Eye Unit

About this book

This book is intended for anyone whose work involves dealing with acute ophthalmic presentations. We have used the term 'practitioner' to include doctors, ophthalmic nurses, emergency care practitioners, nurse practitioners, nurses in accident and emergency departments and 'walk in' centres and first aid workers in remote locations such as oil rigs or working in the armed services. Readers will approach this text with differing levels of confidence, skills and knowledge. We hope this book will help them develop greater competence in ophthalmic emergency practice.

As a slim volume for quick reference, this book cannot include information such as how to put people at ease, ensure confidentiality and care for the specific needs of children, disabled people or other groups with particular needs. We have assumed that any professional given the responsibility of practising care at this level will either already have most of these skills or be seeking other ways to learn and develop them.

The flag system

Throughout this book, we have used a system of flag symbols in the margins to highlight the diagnostic significance of symptoms described in a particular context.

A red flag indicates a highly significant symptom.

An amber flag indicates a symptom that should be treated with caution as a diagnostic tool.

Acknowledgments

The authors wish to acknowledge the contributions of Julie Cartledge, David Goorapah, Helen Storr and Linda Witchell for reading Edition 1 early drafts and making constructive suggestions regarding amendments to the text; Sue Cox for designing the telephone triage form and Sam Hartley for her photography. We would also like to thank Graham Giddens for his help in checking references and for proof reading the second edition. The diagrams in this book have been redrawn, based on originals by Peter Jack in *Ophthalmology for Nurses*, Gaston H., Elkington A., 1986, Croom Helm Publishers.

The authors would like to thank the following for their kind permission to use photographs:

Amanda MacFarlane (front cover photograph)

David Etchells

Eric P. Suan, M.D., F.A.C.S, The Retina Care Center, Baltimore, Maryland, USA

Manchester Royal Eye Hospital, Manchester, UK

The Cogan Collection, National Eye Institute, National Institute of Health, Bethesda, Maryland, USA

Chapter 1
Anatomy and physiology of the eye

This chapter contains some very basic information to get you started. Study of more detailed texts is recommended as your knowledge of this subject grows. A few notes are offered regarding 'clinical significance' to demonstrate the need to apply textbook knowledge to actual eye disorders in order to develop your own understanding of symptoms and treatments.

Protection of the eye

The orbit

Protection of the eye

As a complex, delicate and superficial organ, the eye is reasonably well protected within the bony orbit. The frontal bone of the brow juts out slightly, protecting the eye from many of the larger blunt injuries encountered, such as footballs. This, in combination with the other bones of the orbital rim, maxillary bone and zygomatic bone, makes an exterior protective rim, within which the eye sits. Blunt injuries may result in orbital rim fractures. Orbital fat pads out the available space around the eye, the external muscles of the eye, blood vessels and nerves, and acts as a 'shock absorber' in the event of a direct or indirect impact in the orbital region.

A 'blow out fracture' most commonly affects the orbital floor, the superior aspect of the maxillary bone, but the ethmoid bone, which forms the medial wall of the orbit, is sometimes also involved.

Clinical significance

Eye departments and ophthalmologists are concerned with the function of the eye itself. Although they do see patients with orbital fractures, their remit is primarily the health and function of the eye itself. Other specialisms take responsibility for the management of head injuries and orbital fractures, having consulted the ophthalmologist regarding possible associated eye trauma.

Occasionally an infection spreads to the tissues surrounding the eye, within the orbit (orbital cellulitis), which may be managed either by the ophthalmology or Ear, Nose and Throat (ENT) departments, depending on whether the infection arose from the structures immediately surrounding the eye or from the facial sinuses.

The eyelids

These comprise the next protective structure for the eye. The eyelids close reflexively when a threat is perceived, and the cilia (eyelashes), when touched, will also cause the eye to close rapidly. The skin covering the eyelids is loose and thin and readily accommodates considerable rapid swelling of the eyelid tissue in response to allergy or injury.

Figure 1.1

The eyelid

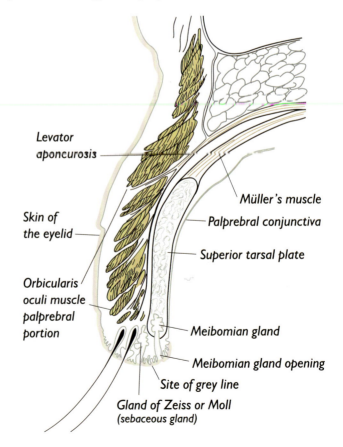

Levator aponeurosis

Müller's muscle

Skin of the eyelid

Palprebral conjunctiva

Superior tarsal plate

Orbicularis oculi muscle palprebral portion

Meibomian gland

Meibomian gland opening

Site of grey line

Gland of Zeiss or Moll (sebaceous gland)

Muscles of the eyelids

The *orbicularis oculi* muscle has three functions.

- It is a sphincter muscle which firmly closes the eyelids, and is particularly efficient in young children. Indeed, a baby squeezing the eyelids shut whilst a practitioner is struggling hard to open them, can cause the upper eyelid to evert spontaneously.
- The blink function of the orbicularis muscle ensures the frequent and even distribution of tears across the eye.
- The slightly lateral action of the muscle across the eye helps to draw small quantities of tears from the lacrimal gland and closure of the eyelids by the orbicularis muscle helps to suck excess tears into the lacrimal punctae.

The *frontalis* muscle from the forehead, the long levator muscle and the shorter *Müller's* muscle all work together to raise the eyelid.

Within the eyelids

The *glands of Zeiss* are sebaceous and lipid-secreting glands associated with eyelash follicles, the sebum from which contributes to the tear film.

The *glands of Moll* are specialised sweat glands, also associated with eyelash follicles.

The *meibomian glands* are located between the tarsal plates and conjunctiva lining the eyelids and produce sebum and lipids, which also contribute to the tear film of the eye. There are about 30 of these glands in the upper eyelid of each eye, and slightly less in the lower eyelids. Their orifices are visible along the margins of the eyelids when examining the eye with a slit lamp. They can also be seen through the conjunctiva when the eyelid is everted. Meibomian glands can become blocked and infected at any age.

The accessory lacrimal glands of *Krause* and *Wolfring* are situated in the fornices of the upper and lower eyelids.

The *tarsal plates* are composed of dense fibrous tissue and provide support and shape to the eyelids and a fair amount of protection against injury to the eyeball itself. The tarsal plates are larger, half moon shapes in the upper eyelids, and thinner and smaller in the lower eyelids, and of an elliptical shape.

Clinical significance

In a facial palsy, the eye may undergo exposure and dryness or other injury due to the failure of the eyelids to close efficiently. Inadequate eyelid closure may also occur as a result of growths on the eyelids, injuries to the eyelids or unskilled eyelid surgery.

The conjunctiva

Figure 1.2

Conjunctival fornices

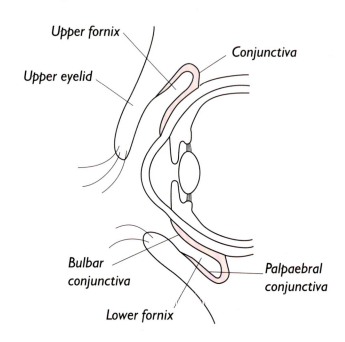

The conjunctiva

The conjunctiva is a thin, transparent mucous membrane that lines the eyelids (known as the palpaebral conjunctiva) and folds back on itself to make the upper and lower fornices. These fornices, or 'pockets' are significant in that loose foreign bodies and misplaced contact lenses are never completely irrecoverable.

The conjunctiva is loosely attached to the anterior part of the sclera (this section is called the bulbar conjunctiva) until it reaches the cornea. The bulbar conjunctiva contains goblet cells, which secrete mucin, an important constituent of the tear film. The very loose attachment of the conjunctiva to the globe makes it an area that can become swollen – conjunctival chemosis – in response to inflammation or allergy. It is also a useful site for subconjunctival injections of antibiotics or steroid drugs to treat some eye conditions.

Anatomy and physiology of the eye

The bulbar conjunctival blood vessels are very fine and are not generally apparent in the normal healthy eye. The conjunctiva ends at the limbus where it merges with the sclera and cornea.
Clinical significance
The appearance of the conjunctiva inside the eyelids and across the front of the globe provides useful diagnostic clues. Scarlet inflammation, primarily inside the eyelids and distal to the cornea, may indicate conjunctivitis. A generalised crimson redness of the conjunctiva, taken together with other critical signs, may indicate an acute ('congestive') glaucoma. Patches of redness, especially of a pinky purple appearance may indicate a problem with the sclera. Scarlet areas of dilated blood vessels may develop distal to a corneal problem such as an ulcer or foreign body. Tiny pinky purple inflamed vessels around the edge of the cornea may indicate an anterior uveitis or keratitis.

Similarly the quality and appearance of any discharge from the conjunctiva needs to be noted and evaluated as a diagnostic step. See the differential diagnostic guides for acute red eye (in 'The conjunctiva', page 28) and types of conjunctivitis (page 129).

The lacrimal apparatus

Figure 1.3
Lacrimal apparatus

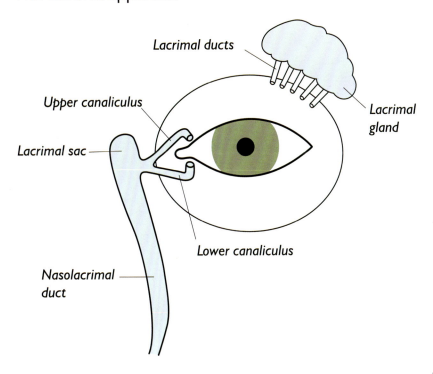

Lacrimal ducts

Upper canaliculus

Lacrimal gland

Lacrimal sac

Lower canaliculus

Nasolacrimal duct

The lacrimal gland

This is about the size and shape of an almond, located at the upper temporal side of each eye, within the lacrimal fossa of the frontal bone of the skull. It has a row of tiny openings which discharge tears across the front of the eye, assisted by the blinking actions of the eyelids. It is, however, the accessory lacrimal glands of Krause and Wolfring which supply the general contribution to the aqueous layer of the tear film. The lacrimal gland produces larger, immediate quantities of tears in response to foreign bodies or chemicals, trauma and disruption of the cornea and emotional upsets.

The blinking actions of the eyelids, combined with gravity, cause the tears to be swept down across the front of the eye towards the upper and lower punctae in the nasal corners of each eye, through the upper and lower canaliculi into the common canaliculus, and from there into the lacrimal sac, through the nasolacrimal duct and into the nose.

Clinical significance

Disorders of either the production or drainage of tears can be inconvenient and at worst potentially damaging to eye health.

The tear film

Figure 1.4

Tear film

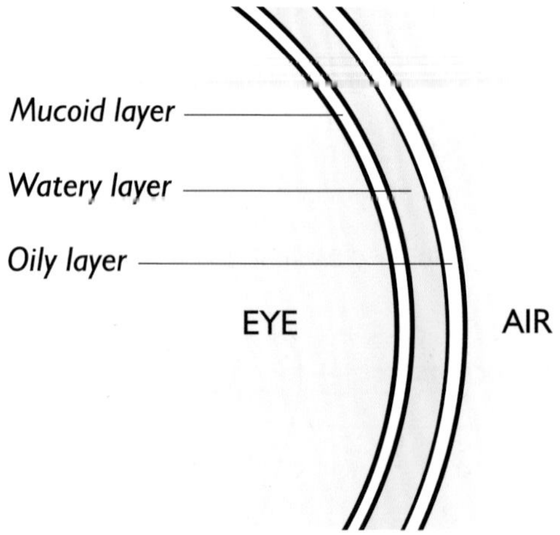

Mucoid layer

Watery layer

Oily layer

EYE   AIR

The tear film has four main functions:
* to prevent the cornea from drying out
* to convey nutrients and oxygen to the cornea as it has no direct blood supply
* to keep the cornea clean and to protect this smooth refractive surface of the eye
* to provide protection against infection.

Anatomy and physiology of the eye

The healthy tear film is complex, consisting of three layers. *Mucin*, the innermost layer, secreted by the goblet cells of the bulbar conjunctiva, clings effectively to the corneal epithelium and its hydrophilic (water attracting) property enables the aqueous (watery) layer to be retained on the surface of the eye.

Aqueous humour, the middle layer of the tear film, is secreted by the glands of Krause and Wolfring. This watery layer contains lysozyme, an enzyme which also occurs in nasal secretions and gastric juices, which has a cytoprotective and bacteriostatic action against a range of pathogens (Fleiszig *et al.* 2003, Minjian *et al.* 2005).

The *lipid* (oily) layer, supplied by the meibomian glands and the glands of Zeiss inhibits evaporation of the tear film, and helps to retain the aqueous on the surface of the eye.

Clinical significance

Given the different areas that produce the components of the tear film, it can easily be seen that a problem with any part of the process will lead to a dysfunctional tear film with attendant problems, notably for the cornea. Always discourage patients from making regular use of proprietary eye washing solutions that will wash away the tear film and the protective lysozyme.

The external eye muscles

Figure 1.5

External eye muscles

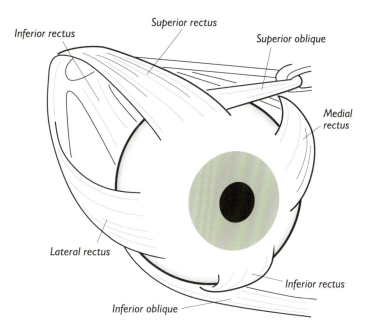

Superior rectus

Inferior rectus

Superior oblique

Medial rectus

Lateral rectus

Inferior rectus

Inferior oblique

Eye Emergencies: The practitioner's guide

There are three pairs of external muscles to move the eyes horizontally, vertically, clockwise and anticlockwise.
Each eye has:

- superior and inferior rectus, lateral and medial rectus
- superior oblique and inferior oblique muscles.

Normally, these muscles move both eyes together in synergy, to produce good binocular vision.

Clinical significance
The external eye muscles need to work efficiently in order for children to develop adequate vision in both eyes (hence a childhood squint sometimes leads to 'lazy eye' in adults), to prevent double vision in adults and to retain a satisfactory cosmetic appearance.

The eye

The eye

The eye itself is sometimes referred to as 'the globe', as in 'ruptured globe' to disassociate it from the other, extra-ocular structures described above.

Figure 1.6

The whole eye

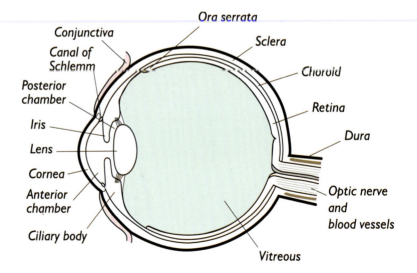

Anatomy and physiology of the eye

The cornea

Figure 1.7

The cornea

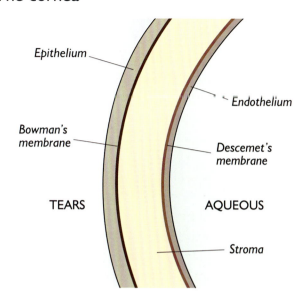

Epithelium

Endothelium

Bowman's membrane

Descemet's membrane

TEARS

AQUEOUS

Stroma

The cornea has three main functions.
- It provides a clear window for light rays to pass through.
- It is responsible for about two-thirds of the eye's refractive power.
- It provides protection for the structures that lie behind it.

The limbus is a transitional area, where the cells of the sclera become rapidly avascular and more transparent, merging into the corneal tissue. The cornea is extremely sensitive, as it contains more nerve endings than anywhere else in the body. It is only about half a millimetre thick and is composed of five layers, listed below from the outermost inwards.
- *Epithelium* – consists of layers of cells with an overall depth of five to six cells. These cells are capable of regeneration if damaged.
- *Bowman's membrane* – is a strong collagen membrane, which, if injured, for example with the removal of a corneal foreign body, will heal as a white scar within a transparent cornea.
- *Corneal stroma* – this represents 90 per cent of the thickness of the cornea. Its lamella sheets are composed of tiny collagen fibrils to give the cornea its clarity. Damage to this also produces white scar tissue.
- *Descemet's membrane* – is the strong, thin elastic basement membrane of the cornea.

- *Endothelium* – is only one cell layer thick, and, once damaged, these cells do not regenerate. The endothelial cells allow nutrients from the aqueous humour to pass into the cornea and actively pump excess fluid from the cornea back into the aqueous.

In recent studies Professor Harminder Dua has detected the presence of a well-defined, acellular, strong layer in the pre-Descemet's cornea (Dua's layer) but as yet little is known about the function and purpose of this layer (Dua *et al.* 2013).

Clinical significance

To function effectively, the cornea must maintain a high level of transparency and in the normal individual is reliant on the tear film on the surface of the eye and the aqueous inside the eye for its nutrition and some of its oxygen needs. The main source of oxygen to the cornea is supplied from the atmosphere. Smoky atmospheres and overuse of contact lenses will therefore inhibit the oxygen supply.

Scarring of the cornea, particularly in the visual axis, will affect visual acuity.

Experienced slit lamp users are able to identify the depth of problems within the cornea, and are therefore better placed to remove rusty corneal foreign bodies, as any work on the cornea with needles and burrs carries a risk of accidental penetration. Their experienced interventions will also cause less corneal scarring.

Figure 1.8

Drainage angle

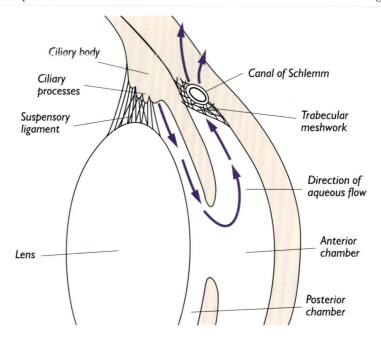

Ciliary body

Ciliary processes

Suspensory ligament

Lens

Canal of Schlemm

Trabecular meshwork

Direction of aqueous flow

Anterior chamber

Posterior chamber

Drainage angle
Aqueous humour
Aqueous humour is secreted by the finger-like structures called ciliary processes, which cover the ciliary body. Its functions are to maintain the shape of the front of the eye, provide nutrition to the cornea and lens and provide a clear pathway for light through the anterior section of the eye. It circulates from the posterior chamber – the small space behind the iris – through the pupil, into the anterior chamber, through the trabecular meshwork, into the canal of Schlemm and thence into the venous system.

Aqueous production and drainage is a process that goes on 24 hours a day, with diurnal peaks and troughs, peaking in the early morning. The amount of aqueous present in the anterior chamber of the average eye is 0.6 ml, and in the posterior chamber is 0.25 ml. According to McKnight *et al.* (2000) the aqueous in the posterior chamber is completely replaced every 30 minutes, and in the anterior chamber every 120 minutes. The intra-ocular pressure at the front of the eye can be measured using a tonometer and average measurements are between 10 and 21 mm Hg.

Clinical significance
The relatively rapid rate of aqueous production and drainage in the normal eye demonstrates how, in an attack of acute glaucoma, the pain accelerates rapidly in about 30 minutes and continues to increase.

Trabecular meshwork
The trabecular meshwork is a circular, spongy network of connective tissue which provides a pressure-sensitive semi-resistant barrier to the outflow of aqueous.

Clinical significance
The trabecular meshwork is one of the ocular mechanisms concerned with regulating the intra-ocular pressure. Bear in mind the possibility of acute blockage of this outflow system as a result of acute glaucoma; debris from intra-ocular surgery; blood cells from bleeding inside the eye; inflammatory cells from auto-immune conditions or intra-ocular infection.

The trabecular meshwork is responsible for the ingestion and digestion of cellular debris and the maintenance of immune privilege in the eye. 'Immune privilege' relates to the fact that the eye can resist most infections without producing inflammation and loss of vision.

The canal of Schlemm is a circular collecting channel at the limbus for aqueous to drain into before absorption by the episcleral veins.

Internal eye muscles

Within the iris there are two muscles that regulate the amount of light entering the eye and have a role in focusing light rays for near and distant vision. They are:

- the *sphincter pupillae*, which constricts the pupil, and
- the *dilator pupillae*, which dilates the pupil.

These muscles are under the control of the nervous system, but can be stimulated or paralysed by eye drops to produce therapeutic or diagnostic pupil mydriasis (dilation) or miosis (constriction).

The large circular *ciliary muscle* within the ciliary body is responsible for altering the thickness of the lens as the major focusing mechanism of the eye and can be paralysed by cycloplegic eye drops for ophthalmic examinations, thus making accommodation for near vision impossible.

The lens

The lens is a transparent biconvex structure, enclosed within a capsular bag which is attached by tiny filamentary suspensory ligaments – the lens zonules – to the ciliary body.

Clinical significance

It is possible for the lens to become dislocated as a result of Marfan's syndrome or trauma. Bear in mind that the lens grows and hardens throughout life, and that by the age of 40 or so it will have lost about half of its previous focusing power, leading to the need for 'reading glasses'. By the age of about 60, there is little focusing power left in the lens. Repeated blunt trauma, for example boxing, will cause a disruption in the continuous growth of the lens fibres causing traumatic cataract. A penetrating injury that damages the lens capsule can cause a disruption in the chemistry inside the lens, resulting in a swollen, cataractous lens within days and sometimes hours of the injury.

The sclera

This tough, white outer coat of the eye provides protection for the more delicate inner layers and acts as an anchor point for the external eye muscles.

The uveal tract

The uveal tract comprises the choroid, the 'middle layer' of the eye, the iris and the ciliary body that are continuous with it. It is affected by inflammatory processes that are variously described as iritis, iridocyclitis, cyclitis, choroiditis, anterior uveitis and posterior uveitis.

The iris

The iris has a genetically determined colour. It regulates the light entering the eye and contributes to the focusing power of the eye. It is attached at its outer border to the sclera and anterior ciliary body.

Clinical significance

As a result of blunt trauma, a section of the iris can be torn from its root (iridodialysis) or its delicate blood vessels may bleed, causing a hyphaema. Iris tissue may prolapse through a penetration of the globe. It is possible for the iris to stick to the underside of the cornea (anterior synaechia) or to the anterior surface of the lens (posterior synaechia) under certain conditions, thereby impeding aqueous drainage.

The ciliary body

The ciliary body has the twin functions of secreting aqueous fluid and providing the attachments for the lens zonules. Contraction and relaxation of the ciliary body changes the focusing power of the lens.

Clinical significance

Cycloplegic eye drops temporarily paralyse the ciliary muscle, which enables experienced ophthalmologists and optometrists to prescribe spectacles for babies and young children. Cycloplegic eye drops also help to reduce the pain of anterior uveitis and prevent posterior synechiae.

The choroid

The choroid contains many blood vessels and is responsible for most of the arterial and venous blood supply to the eye. It contributes to the regulation of the intra-ocular pressure via the uveo-scleral drainage route. The choroid lies in close apposition to the sclera, but is not attached. There is the possibility of a choroid detachment occurring if the pressure in the eye becomes very low, for example after filtration surgery to reduce the eye pressure in people with open angle glaucoma, but the situation resolves naturally once the intra-ocular pressure returns to normal.

The retina

The retina is the innermost layer of the eye, containing the visually sensitive photoreceptors, and the central retinal vein and artery that provide nutrition and waste transport. Images are transmitted from the rod- and cone-shaped photoreceptors, via the optic nerve, to the brain, where they are interpreted. As part of its embryonic development, the retina originally consisted of two layers, a neural layer and a pigmented layer that became fused as the embryo developed.

The macula (sometimes referred to as the 'yellow spot') is a specialised area of the retina, containing many cone cells, which provides our clear, detailed colour vision. The fovea is a depression, located in the centre of the macula, and contains only cone cells for the sharpest possible vision.

Clinical significance

The retina, which arose developmentally from two completely separate layers, can 'detach'. This is when the pigmented layer and the neural layer separate as a result of trauma or medical conditions within the eye. The macula is crucial for clear vision and, if detached, rarely recovers its original sensitivity following successful surgery. The retina is reliant for function on its arterial blood supply and venous drainage, and interruptions to this will cause rapid loss of vision. There are an increasing number of individuals who are suffering from macular degeneration as a result of age-related changes at the back of the eye, which causes loss of central vision or a more complete loss of sight.

Vitreous humour

The vitreous humour is a thick gel-like substance that fills the posterior part of the eye. It is largely water, but its gel consistency is achieved by tiny collagen fibrils. The vitreous is attached at the ora serata, the anterior periphery of the retina, which becomes continuous with the columnar cells of the ciliary body.

Clinical significance

Any sudden loss of vitreous as a result of injury can lead to a retinal detachment, as the acute loss of pressure within the eye will lead to tension on the areas of attachment. The vitreous does tend to shrink over the normal lifetime, and a vitreous detachment may lead to the development of acute visual symptoms, the tearing of a small retinal vessel and subsequent haemorrhage into the vitreous and even to retinal detachment.

The optic pathways

The optic pathways

Most people regard the eye as the organ of sight. Few of the general public appreciate that the eye itself is only a part of a complex mechanism that leads to perception of the world around us. Visual interpretation by the brain is a learned response, which begins on the day of birth and continues until the age of about five to eight. For this reason, it is important that the child has both eyes reasonably straight so that central images fall on the macula. Unless this happens consistently, the brain may 'switch off' an inferior image from a squinting eye. For similar reasons, it is generally considered unwise to cover a child's eye for more than a few hours, unless under orthoptic supervision.

Figure 1.9

The optic pathways

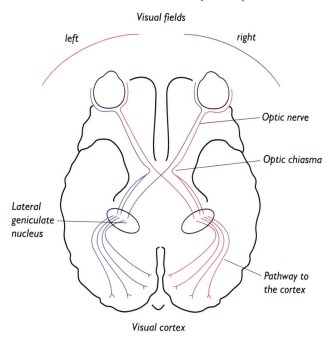

Visual fields

left   right

Optic nerve

Optic chiasma

Lateral geniculate nucleus

Pathway to the cortex

Visual cortex

Eye Emergencies: The practitioner's guide

The *optic nerves* are paired cranial nerves, known also as cranial nerve II. They are considered to be part of the brain system, and are covered as with the brain, by pia, arachnoid and dura mater. Unlike peripheral nerves throughout the body, they do not regenerate if injured or diseased and so damage will result in partial or complete loss of vision.

As may be seen from Figure 1.9, images from the retinae are carried along the optic nerves to the *optic chiasma*, sitting just above the pituitary gland, where the optic nerve fibres carrying visual information from the left and right visual fields partially cross, so that all the information from the right visual field is managed by the left visual system of the brain, and information from the left visual field is processed by the right visual system of the brain.

The *lateral geniculate* nuclei are 'staging posts' in the brain's thalamus where information regarding motion, colour and brightness or darkness is processed.

The *optic radiations* connect the lateral geniculate nuclei with the visual cortex in the occipital lobe of the brain, where vision is interpreted in five areas.

Clinical significance

Damage to any part of the visual pathway will result in a loss of visual perception in a recognisable pattern which will give the neurologist indications regarding the area of the brain which has been damaged. Neurologists and ophthalmologists often work together on these problems, as the ophthalmic department has specialised equipment for charting the visual fields, but this is not primarily an ophthalmic problem. The public sometimes have difficulty understanding the relationship between vision and brain function.

References

Dua, H.S., Faraj, L.A., Said, D.G., Gray, T. and Lowe, J. (2013). Human corneal anatomy redefined: a novel pre-Descemet's layer (Dua's layer). *Ophthalmology*, 120(9): 1778–1785.

Fleiszig, S., Kwong, M. and Evans, D. (2003). Modification of Pseudomonas Aeruginosa interactions with corneal epithelial cells by human tear fluid. *Infection and Immunology*, 71(7): 3866–3874.

McKnight, A., McLaughlin, C., Peart, D., Purves, R., Carre, D. and Civan M. (2000). *Clinical and Experimental Pharmacology and Physiology*, 27(1–2): 100.

Minjian, N., Evans, D., Hawgood, S., Anders, E., Sack, R. and Fleiszig, S. (2005). Surfactant Protein D is present in human tear fluid and the cornea and inhibits epithelial cell invasion by Pseudomonas aeruginosa. *Infection and Immunity*, 73(4): 2147–2156.

Chapter 2
Initial assessment

Ophthalmic triage

Ophthalmic triage

Triage is an effective way of gathering information from the patient and making a decision about how urgently the patient needs to be seen. It is also an opportunity to give the patient education and advice about their condition and any information about immediate care needs. Telephone triage has become mainstream in many ophthalmic Emergency Departments and presents challenges in that the patient is not assessed face to face.

Triage is designed to be a fast initial assessment of the patient to decide on clinical priority (Marsden 2006). In 2000 Marsden described ophthalmic telephone triage as 'gathering information by questioning the patient or healthcare professional about the perceived problem and making decisions as to the most appropriate form of management' (Marsden 2000). There has been much debate about the benefits of telephone triage, particularly since the introduction of NHS Direct in 1998. This generated an array of literature examining the system, all now fairly dated. However the general consensus appears to be that if it is guided by protocols, and health professionals are well educated, then it is a safe and effective method of managing patient care based on the urgency of need (Bunn *et al.* 2005).

Marsden (2006) believes that telephone triage should be undertaken by experienced practitioners and works well when it is carried out correctly. This relies on good training of competent practitioners. Ring and Linnell (2008) described an initiative to improve services in an ophthalmic Emergency Department, introducing a formal triage tool to aid decision-making and reduce the risk of inappropriate patient management.

The ophthalmic nurse-led triage process

(via telephone or face to face):

- summarises pertinent information from the patient
- decides on the most appropriate care pathway for the patient
  – ophthalmologist, ophthalmic nurse, primary physician, optometrist or community pharmacist
- if an ophthalmic review is required, decides on the degree of urgency
- provides the patient with information, education and reassurance
- provides documented records for subsequent queries and audits.

(See Chapter 8 for an example Record of Telephone Triage Advice – Eye Unit and a Patient Assessment – Eye Accident and Emergency telephone triage tool.)

Good ophthalmic triage by experienced ophthalmic nurses has contributed effectively to raising the standards of patient care in many areas of the NHS. It has the potential to avoid unnecessary attendances for elderly or incapacitated people, save travel costs associated with patient attendance and save time for busy, stressed patients. In turn, this has released time in hectic NHS departments to spend on patients whose eye conditions are unsuitable for self-care or management within the community.

If you work within a primary care setting, acquaint yourself with and make use of any existing local ophthalmic triage arrangements. There are times when you should refer a patient immediately after first aid treatment, for example in the case of severe chemical injury. Guidance in this and subsequent chapters should help you and hospital-based ophthalmic staff to reach careful, reasoned decisions, supported by good documentation.

There are three procedures which will help the practitioner to reach a reasonable provisional diagnosis of an eye condition. The first is to record a thorough ophthalmic history, either personally or by telephone triage. The second is to test the patient's central visual acuity and the third is to make a pen torch examination of both eyes.

Recording an 'eye' history

Recording an 'eye' history

General advice

Key points to remember when recording an 'eye' history face to face, or by telephone, include the following:

- If information is being gathered from a patient on your premises, ensure privacy and confidentiality.
- Ask the patient why they have contacted you. Listen very carefully to what they tell you. Ask questions as appropriate. Ask them to clarify their meaning if necessary. Never ask leading questions or put words into their mouths.
- Ask what the eye symptoms are, when the patient noticed them and what they were doing immediately beforehand (particularly if the onset of symptoms is sudden).

It may be helpful to record the visual acuity in both eyes at this stage. If it is a telephone consultation, ask them to cover one eye at a time, and look at the clock, a book or magazine and try to estimate whether there has been any recent change in the vision of either eye. The only occasions when you don't test the vision first are:

  - when the patient is seriously ill, and you need to assess the general condition first, or
  - when the patient is suffering from a chemical injury and you need to treat this first.

- Always note and record whether the patient has a history of doing any dangerous work, such as hammering, or using power tools, and ask whether they were wearing any eye protection. If they were near an explosion without eye protection they are at increased risk of getting intra-ocular foreign bodies. Check their occupation. This may give a clue as to the problem.
- Ask about any previous eye problems. This may give valuable clues, particularly if there is a history of poor vision in one eye at birth or the possible recurrence of previous eye disease, notably inflammatory problems.
- Ask about any family history of eye problems. Some problems, for example the tendency to develop cataract, retinal detachment and open angle glaucoma, may be inherited.

- Ask about any general illnesses. For example, some conditions, such as inflammatory bowel disease and rheumatoid type conditions, are known to be linked to inflammatory eye problems. Is there, or has there been any recent illness? A cold or flu might indicate a viral eye condition.

- Ask about any tablets or medicines being taken. This history will provide further information about known medical problems which may have a bearing on the eye complaint. For example, hypertension may be associated with some vascular eye diseases such as central retinal vein occlusion; diabetes may give rise to diabetic retinopathy; systemic inflammatory disease, for example sarcoidosis, may give rise to ocular inflammation.

- Record any allergies precisely. This may have a bearing on allergic eye conditions influencing your choice of treatment. Lanolin allergies need to be documented as some eye ointments use lanolin as the carrier for the active constituents.

- Record pain level and type. Be very accurate with this, using a pain scale. Ask detailed questions about the exact type of pain and location. Ask whether they have taken any analgesia and whether it helped. Record the type of pain, and discriminate between irritation, stinging and soreness. Look out for photophobia, deep pain in and around the eye and severe eye pain, particularly when associated with nausea and vomiting.

- Age may be significant, as certain eye problems may affect particular age groups; for example, circulatory problems and macular degeneration generally occur in older people.

If conducting telephone triage remember also to:

- note the patient's name and telephone number first, just in case you need to ring back
- always document the date and time of telephone conversations. You will then have an *aide memoire* should questions be asked later, or if a complaint is made
- make every effort to speak to the patient personally, rather than taking secondhand information from a caller.

Vision testing

Basic equipment

- Snellen or LogMAR test chart
- Sheridan Gardiner test chart
- Pinhole occluder.

Testing visual acuity

Testing visual acuity is one of the most important aids to diagnosis in ophthalmology and is carried out every time a patient visits for eye treatment in order to assess progress or deterioration. It is not a legal requirement but it could be useful to you if a patient were ever to try to make a claim against you.

If you are unable to use a Snellen chart, perhaps on home visits, consider the possibility of using a Sheridan Gardiner test.

The Snellen chart

Although many ophthalmic departments now use LogMAR vision testing, the Snellen chart is still used widely and displays standard letters in decreasing sizes. This provides a well-recognised measurement of central visual acuity. The letters are numbered from 60 at the top, down to four or five at the bottom, and are printed in black on a white background. The chart should be well lit for test purposes.

Check the size of the chart you have. The full-sized chart is designed to be read at a distance of six metres. In a small space, this can be 'doubled' by the use of an appropriate mirror at three metres. It is also possible to obtain 'reduced' charts to be read at three metres.

How to test

Vision testing should be carried out in a private area. The patient should not be distracted, interrupted or embarrassed.

Position the patient six metres away from the chart and note whether they are wearing contact lenses. Make sure that they put on their bifocals or distance spectacles if they have them. If the patient is confused about 'distance glasses' ask them whether they wear spectacles for driving or watching television, and, if so, to put these on. Ask the patient to gently cover one eye at a time, with a cupped hand (or you can use a disinfected occluder) and to read out what they can see. Make sure that each eye is properly covered throughout the test of the other eye.

The result for a person with average (or corrected) eyesight is usually 6/6.

In this case, the 6 at the top of the fraction is the number of metres the patient was sitting away from the chart. The bottom 6 is the size of letters the person with average sight would be able to see when six metres away from the chart.

Eye Emergencies: The practitioner's guide

Suppose, however, that a very myopic (short-sighted) person without spectacles was only able to read the large letter at the top of the chart. The vision would be recorded as 6/60. The top figure is still 6, because the person is still six metres away from the chart. The bottom figure is now 60, denoting that this person is only able to see what the average person (with 6/6 vision) would be able to see from a distance of 60 metres from the chart. (Each line on the chart is labelled with a tiny number underneath to indicate the distance at which the letters can be read by an average-sighted person.)

Always remember, when you are recording a person's vision, to state whether the test was carried out wearing spectacles or contact lenses (aided) or not (unaided).

The results of the Visual Acuity Test are written as follows:

Right Visual Acuity	Left Visual Acuity
6/12	6/18
(unaided)	
6/6	6/9
(with spectacles or contact lenses)	

A person with perfectly healthy eyes may only be able to see, for example, 6/12 without spectacles but manage to read as far as the 6/4 line with spectacles or contact lenses. To conserve time, it is normal for the emergency practitioner to test the person's sight just once, with the patient wearing their distance spectacles or bifocals. *Note:* Children don't like to get tests 'wrong'. If you are using a Snellen chart, turn the chart to a fresh set of letters for the second eye, in case the first set has been memorised.

Pinhole

Visual acuity at 6/12 or lower is also measured through a pinhole, to see whether a person needs spectacles or the low visual acuity results from injury or disease. In a person who would benefit from spectacles, use of a pinhole will increase the visual acuity by two lines or more.

The pinhole is also useful for testing the person who wears distance spectacles but has not got them with them.

If the patient's pupil has been dilated, the lens in the eye may be less able to accommodate and the vision may be reduced as a result. Check with a pinhole to see whether this makes any improvement. Record your findings.

If you don't have a pinhole, make one for single use quickly, using a circle of cardboard from the lid of a box of paper tissues. Make a small hole with an injection needle. If there is no improvement in the vision with use of a pinhole, this is likely to indicate a pathological problem.

Visual acuity is then recorded:

[right eye]	[left eye]
RVA 6/6 with glasses	LVA CF
	LVA 6/12 (PH)

The LogMAR chart

LogMAR is an algorithm for the logarithm of the minimum angle of resolution (MAR). The distance visual acuity of patients assessed using a logMAR chart is expressed as a logarithmic value. Put another way, the smaller the letters on the chart, and the further they are away, the smaller the value of the logMAR score associated with it.

LogMAR charts 'crowd' the letters together, rather like printed documents, and are thus felt to provide more accurate results (Reid 2006). The patient is asked to read along the letters, starting with the larger ones at the top of the chart. A score is given for each letter that is read correctly. As with the Snellen test, they are encouraged to guess, and the test is stopped when four mistakes are made in one line. This test is now regularly used in macular degeneration clinics where it is felt that the acuity score may help to detect subtle changes in vision.

Count fingers

When a patient is unable to see letters on the board, a hand with outstretched fingers is held in front of the patient and the distance recorded at which the fingers can be successfully counted (CF at 1 m or CF at 0.5 m).

Hand movements

If the patient can't manage to count fingers, check whether they can see a hand waving in front of them. This is recorded as hand movements (HM). Check in all quadrants of vision as the patient may also have large visual field defects.

Perception of light

Finally, check whether or not the patient can perceive light (PL or

NPL) in response to flashes from a pen torch in the four quadrants of vision.

Abbreviations used for records

PH	Pinhole
VA	Visual acuity
CF	Count fingers
HM	Hand movements
PL	Perception of light
NPL	No perception of light
Glss	Glasses
U/A	Vision was tested without glasses
AE	Artificial eye
CL	Contact lenses

'Lazy eye' (amblyopic eye)

Occasionally you will meet a patient who has one eye 'weaker' than the other. They may state that they were treated for 'squint' in childhood. Because at one stage the eye was misaligned, and still might be, the brain never received a clear image on this side, and visual perception did not develop as well as it might have done. Surgery may have been carried out for cosmetic appearance in adults but will not alter or improve the vision. There is no treatment for this in the adult, and you should document this information:

> 6/12 *(patient says lazy eye)*

Driving vision

Visual field defects need to be assessed in a hospital ophthalmic out-patient department according to the classes of vehicles specified in the individual's driving licence. DVLA (2015) also requires the reading of a standard number plate in good lighting conditions at 20 metres. This requirement is absolute in law. This equates to reading vision of 6/12 on a Snellen chart. You should inform the patient if their eyesight may not reach the driving standard and suggest that they go for a check with an optometrist once their acute eye condition has settled.

The Sheridan Gardiner test for children

This is useful for a child who can recognise letters by shape but is unable to say what they are. It is also useful for testing people with learning difficulties and non-English speakers. It is also less confusing and quicker for people under the influence of alcohol or drugs to show them just one letter at a time. You must always make a note that the Sheridan Gardiner test was used, as results may differ slightly from the Snellen test. (You must also always ensure privacy for adults using this test.)

A card with one letter on it is held six metres away. In the case of a child, the child sits, with one eye covered, on an adult's knee, holding a card and is asked to point to the corresponding letter from a choice of six or eight. The adult confirms whether they have chosen the correct letter.

As with Snellen testing, ensure privacy and minimise distractions for a child. The eye unit's orthoptic department may be able to help with establishing the level of visual acuity with a pre-verbal or unco-operative child or a baby.

Unless local guidelines state differently, patients with loss or decrease in visual acuity within the previous 24 hours should be discussed with an ophthalmologist urgently (even in the middle of the night). If the change occurred less than a week ago, the ophthalmologist must be consulted promptly the next day.

R. S. V. P.

Remember, you need to urgently evaluate the eye if:

- Red
- Sensitive to light
- Vision is 'down'
- Painful.

The information on the following pages will help you to do this.

Basic eye examination kit

- Good light source – angle poise lamp or pen torch (with a cobalt blue filter if possible)
- Magnification – ideally, in minor injuries or general ED departments, where a slit lamp is not available, obtain a binocular headband magnifier for the department. If you have not yet purchased a binocular magnifier, use your reading glasses if you are long-sighted. Short-sighted people sometimes take their spectacles off to improve their near vision.
- Hand-held (direct) ophthalmoscope – helpful if you can use one.

These are more often used in primary care settings. Ophthalmologists and nurses in advanced ophthalmic practice tend to use hand-held lenses with the slit lamp and the indirect ophthalmoscope.

- Box of paper tissues
- Cotton wool buds
- Fluorescein eye drops, saline eye drops, local anaesthetic drops – Oxybuprocaine is the best for general purposes. Proxymetacaine is said to sting less, and, if you have it available, is considered better for children.

Eye examination with a pen torch

If you have a direct ophthalmoscope available, remember that the slit of light can, if used carefully, give a reasonable magnification of external eye structures such as the eyelid margins, conjunctiva and cornea. You will need a pen torch with a cobalt blue filter for the best results if you intend to use fluorescein. (The green filter on your ophthalmoscope is only used for examining red blood vessels in fine detail; it doesn't work with fluorescein.)

General evaluation and management

- Carefully glance at the patient and note possible clues which may influence your communication with them such as fear, anger or possible depression.
- Look for factors such as nutritional status, age, mobility, cleanliness, fever and pallor which may give diagnostic clues.
- Always allow extra time for children and frightened patients, remembering that it is vital to provide effective reassurance in order to gain the co-operation you will need to examine for, and possibly treat, an eye condition.
- Useful opportunities may arise to give health advice such as reminding patients to use protective equipment to avoid future eye injuries, stressing the importance of good diet for corneal healing and health and suggesting ways to avoid spreading conjunctivitis to others in a family.

The face

Examine the face for:

- swelling – this could indicate preseptal or orbital cellulitis

- bruising
- burns
- cuts
 ● protruding foreign bodies
- abrasions
- rashes
- a swollen pre-auricular gland which may indicate a viral infection.
 ● a protruding eye (proptosis), if this is abnormal for the patient.

The eyelids

Examine the eyelids for the following symptoms.

- Cuts – these often require specialist suturing. Full thickness lacerations may indicate a penetration of the eye.
- Swollen eyelids. As you assess them, remember that orbital cellulitis is potentially fatal. If you suspect this, refer immediately, even in the middle of the night.
- Ingrowing eyelashes, lice infestations on eyelashes
- Small swellings, e.g. styes and cysts
- 'Growths', e.g. papillomas, potential basal cell carcinomas
- Blepharitis
- Discharge
- Eyelids turning in (entropion) or out (ectropion). Both these conditions need routine ophthalmic outpatient referral.
- Foreign bodies inside upper and lower lids
- Look inside the lids for follicles, papillae, concretions.

  Follicles – raised, rounded, avascular white/grey structures containing collections of lymphocytes, found usually in the conjunctiva lining the lower eyelid and the border of the upper tarsal plate. They are frequently noted in viral and chlamydial infections.

  Papillae – tiny raised structures, tightly packed together, containing blood vessels. Many tiny papillae packed together produce a velvety red appearance to the conjunctiva inside the eyelids, typical of bacterial conjunctivitis. Papillae may mass together to form larger lesions, pale red in colour (cobblestones), as in giant papillary conjunctivitis or vernal catarrh. Papillae are a non-specific sign of conjunctival inflammation or allergy.

  Concretions – tiny, creamy/white irregular inclusion cysts embedded within the conjunctiva.

Eye Emergencies: The practitioner's guide

The conjunctiva

Examine the conjunctiva for:

 • subconjunctival haemorrhage, cuts, abrasions – if associated with trauma these may indicate a small penetrating injury

• dilated blood vessels – note whether these are inside the eyelids or overlying the sclera

 • dilated blood vessels around the cornea – known as a ciliary flush – indicative of uveitis

 • conjunctival ischaemia following chemical injury

• a dusky, generally red eye, along with the other acute signs, accompanies an acute glaucoma.

Conjunctivitis is probably the most common, but least serious, cause of a red eye. (See differential diagnosis guide for acute red eye on page 33.) If the vision is normal in both eyes, the cornea bright, the redness is mainly inside the eyelids, appears beefy red, and the eye(s) are sticky, this may be the problem. Purulent (creamy/white) or mucopurulent (yellowish) exudate indicates a bacterial infection. Serous discharge, watery or yellow-tinged, suggests viral infection. Scanty, stringy discharge sometimes occurs in allergic conditions.

The cornea

Examine the cornea for:

• contact lenses – never instil fluorescein unless these are removed, as soft lenses will permanently absorb the stain

 • a dull, hazy cornea – a sudden rise in intra-ocular pressure will cause a hazy cornea, symptomatic of acute glaucoma

• any blood vessels encroaching on to the cornea (can indicate e.g. contact lens over-wear)

• obvious opacities – possibly indicative of old trauma if this accords with history, otherwise possibly something acute, e.g. a twig brushed the front of the eye

 • embedded foreign bodies

 • green stain in a fluorescein test – denotes diseased or injured epithelium

 • a potential full thickness laceration or a pseudomonas ulcer in a contact lens wearer. (See 'Major eye injuries' in Chapter 3 and 'Corneal infections' in Chapter 4.)

Eye movements

Check for eye movements and double vision in all positions of gaze and chart (see 'Visual perception disorders' in Chapter 4 and 'Checking eye movements' in Chapter 9) and check for any pain on eye movements.

 Sudden or recent eye movement disorders are cause for concern but most can wait for normal daytime consultation and the ophthalmologist will generally see them within 24 hours. If they are accompanied by eyelid droop, headache and a dilated pupil, refer immediately as this may be indicative of a potentially fatal neurological condition.

The iris

Check the colour of the iris, which should normally correspond with that of the other eye. Heterochromia describes irises which are not matching in colour. This may be present at birth, with no other eye abnormality.

Heterochromic iris may also result from:

- raised intra-ocular pressure in acute glaucoma
- uveitis
- rubeosis iridis
- Fuchs heterochromic cyclitis
- use of Latanoprost (Xalatan), Travoprost (Travatan), Tafluprost (Saflutan) or Bimatoprost (Lumigan)– this will alter the iris colour, and, if used for one eye only in those with mixed colour irides, brown pigmentation will develop, causing heterochromia.

Check the shape of the iris. A 'peaked' pupil may indicate a leaking anterior chamber, where the iris has flowed out of a wound and effectively plugged it. Sometimes, as a result of blunt trauma, the iris has been torn at the periphery and the pupil looks D-shaped.

The pupil

The pupil is the black area in the centre of the iris which relaxes and contracts to control the amount of light reaching the retina. Normally it responds to:

light – as light increases, the parasympathetic nervous system contracts the spincter pupillae muscle inside the iris to miose (contract) the pupil. The dilator pupillae muscle of the iris, under the control of the sympathetic nervous system, dilates the pupil under low lighting conditions.

close focusing – the 'near' response. When a person looks at a near object, the eyes focus (accommodation) as the ciliary muscle contracts to increase the power of the lens. The pupils reduce in size as the focusing power of the eyes is increased. This process also causes the eyes to turn slightly inwards (converge), so that the near images received by each eye are focused accurately on the most sensitive area of the retina, the fovea.

psychological stimuli – the psychological response (sympathetic nervous system). Fear will cause the pupil to enlarge.

drugs – eye drops may be used for examination purposes, or therapeutically, to miose (reduce pupil size) or to cause mydriasis (an increase in pupil size) (see 'Pupil dilators' in Chapter 6). Misuse of some drugs will similarly produce mydriasis – stimulants such as cocaine and amphetamines, and hallucinogenics such as LSD and mescaline, cause extremely dilated pupils. Narcotics such as heroin, codeine, morphine, or pethidine cause miosis. Responses to therapeutic drugs need to be borne in mind with reference to precipitating acute glaucoma. Some travel sickness prevention medications contain hyoscine, which causes some pupil dilation. Similarly, atropine used peri-operatively will also cause pupil dilation.

Examining pupil reflexes

Are the pupils equal and reacting normally? Anisocoria is the technical term to refer to a difference in pupil sizes which may be traumatic, due to a medical disorder, drug induced or peculiar to the individual (idiopathic).

- A small pupil – the pupil of an eye with uveitis is usually smaller due to reflex spasm of the iris spincter muscle. If accompanied by photophobia, this is an indicator for iritis.

- A mid-dilated, oval pupil not reacting to light is characteristic of acute glaucoma.

- An oddly shaped pupil – evaluate this in conjunction with any past ophthalmic history, particularly injury.

Relative afferent pupillary defect (RAPD)

 Always check for this for before dilating for further examination. (See Chapter 9.)

Check the anterior chamber for:

 ● flat anterior chamber (indicates penetration or post-surgical leak)

 ● obvious intra-ocular foreign bodies, hypopyon (pus in the anterior chamber) or hyphaema (blood in the anterior chamber).

Based on the history, visual acuity and pen torch examination above, you should now be formulating an initial diagnosis, and deciding whether you will treat or refer this patient.

Slit lamp examination

If you are able to carry out a slit lamp examination, working on the pro forma above, it will provide more detailed information. Small lesions on the eyelids can be evaluated, meibomianitis detected, the depth of corneal abrasions estimated and the anterior chamber thoroughly examined.

Check for inflammatory cells in the aqueous by looking in the oblique slit lamp beam under maximum intensity and magnification. The beam should be 2 mm long and 1 mm wide and the cells are seen as tiny particles moving slowly through the tiny beam of light. Kanski and Bowling (2011) suggests that cells should be measured as follows.

The examiner counts the number of cells they can see in the slit lamp beam.

Grade	Cells in field
0	< 1
+/-	1–5
1 +	6–15
2 +	16–25
3 +	26–50
4 +	> 50

Aqueous flare is an inflammatory haze in the aqueous. Kanski and Bowling (2011) similarly advises grading of aqueous flare as follows.

Grade	Description
0	Nil
1 +	Just detectable

2 +	Moderate (iris and lens details clear)
3 +	Marked (iris and lens details hazy)
4 +	Intense (fibrinous exudates)

Record and evaluate all deviations.

As you begin to make a provisional diagnosis, refer to other sections of this book for further diagnostic and treatment advice.

References

British National Formulary 2014
Available at https://www.medicinescomplete.com (accessed 10.02.15).

Bunn, F., Byrne, G. and Kendall, S. (2005). The effects of telephone consultation and triage on healthcare use and patient satisfaction: a systematic review. *British Journal of General Practice*, 55(521): 956–961.

DVLA 2015. *Visual Disorders. Medical Rules.* London DVLA.
Available at https://www.gov.uk/driving-eyesight-rules (accessed 10.02.15).

Kanski, J. and Bowling, B. (2011). *Clinical Ophthalmology: A Systematic Approach.* 7th Ed. Philadelphia PA: Elsevier Limited.

Marsden, J. (2000). *Telephone Triage in an Ophthalmic ED Department.* London: Whurr Publishers Ltd.

Marsden, J. (2006). *Ophthalmic Care.* Chichester: Whurr Publishers Ltd.

Reid, L. (2006). Functional Assessment of Vision. Scottish Sensory Centre.
Available at: http://www.ssc.education.ed.ac.uk/courses/vi&multi/vmay06a.html

Ring, L. and Linnell, A. (2008). Streamlining a specialist A&E service to enhance patient care. *Nursing Times*, 104(26): 29–30.

Differential diagnostic guide: acute red eyes

SIGN/SYMPTOM	CONJUNCTIVITIS	ACUTE UVEITIS	KERATITIS	ACUTE GLAUCOMA
ONSET	Gradual	Slow	Slow	Acute, within 30 minutes
VISUAL ACUITY	Normal	May decrease as condition progresses	May decrease as condition progresses	Speedily severely reduced
PAIN	Gritty, irritable, itchy, possible foreign body sensation	Moderate ache	Moderate pain	Moderate to unbearable, radiating around orbit
PHOTOPHOBIA	No	Moderate/severe	Moderate/severe	Moderate
DISCHARGE	Depends on type	Watery eye	Watery/sticky	Reflex watering
EYELIDS	Possible mild swelling/redness Sticky lashes	Normal	Normal, possibly slightly red	Fairly normal
CONJUNCTIVA	Scarlet red, mainly inside eyelids	Red around the cornea	Red around the cornea	Diffuse dull crimson red
CORNEA	Bright and clear Sometimes punctate staining	Sometimes keratic precipitates* (cells on back of cornea)	Cloudy Ulcerated	Hazy Corneal oedema
ANTERIOR CHAMBER	Clear	Cells and flare	Flare or hypopyon	Shallow, poor view
IRIS	Normal	Muddy	May be muddy	Greenish
PUPIL	Normal	Pupil opening may be irregular from adhesions	Normal	Oval, semi-dilated
REACTION TO LIGHT	Normal	Sluggish	Normal	Unreacting
PRESSURE	Normal	Normal but possible moderate dip or rise	Normal	Raised Hard to palpation
SYSTEMIC SYMPTOMS	Recent cold/hayfever/ asthma Enlarged pre-auricular gland	Possible systemic inflammatory disease	Possible herpes zoster/herpes simplex	Vomiting Possible abdominal symptoms

Eye Emergencies: The practitioner's guide

Visual disturbance assessment chart

DIAGNOSIS	PATHOLOGY	SIGNS AND SYMPTOMS	ACTION	FURTHER INFORMATION
TIA (Transient Ischaemic Attack)	Acute, temporary, neurologic dysfunction as a result of ischaemia	Symptoms generally last less than one hour but can be apparent for 24 hours and resolve completely. Contributory factors can include recent surgery, previous stroke, co-morbidities, e.g. diabetes or cardiovascular disease can occur following blunt or torsion injury to the neck. Check for changes in behaviour, speech, gait, memory, and movement.	If the patient phones with TIA symptoms they must be advised to contact their GP ASAP – a letter should be faxed to their GP informing them of this. Trusts may have a walk-in TIA clinic or immediate referral – check local protocol. If not then give them a TIA letter and advise them to see their GP. Document this on initial assessment.	Standard GP referral letter for TIA is useful. Or there may be standard TIA referral documentation.
CVA/Stroke	The sudden loss of circulation to an area of the brain. Can be ischaemic (caused by emboli or thrombosis) or haemorrhagic in nature (those with haemorrhagic strokes tend to be more poorly).	Ischaemic CVA can present with any of the following: complete or partial hemianopia, monocular or binocular visual loss, diplopia, reduced co-ordination, one sided weakness or paralysis, aphasia. History of cardiovascular disorders, diabetes, and hypertension can be relevant. Haemorrhagic strokes may be more likely to report headache, nausea and vomiting.	Needs urgent medical review (if new symptoms). Patient should be directed to A&E. NICE Guidelines state: ● All patients with suspected stroke should be tested with the FAST (Face Arm Speech Test) or similar test to recognise symptoms of acute stroke. ● All patients with acute stroke should be taken to hospital as quickly as possible and transferred from A&E to an acute stroke unit ● High-risk patients who have already had a TIA should receive a diagnosis, investigations and initial treatment within 24 hours.	One point to note is that patients who have subarachnoid haemorrhage may have sudden onset headache, with neck stiffness, photophobia and pain on ocular movements, nausea and vomiting.
Amaurosis fugax	A symptom of carotid artery disease, small fragments of plaque which have built up in the artery break free and block the retinal artery; the visual disturbance lasts as long as the blockage is present.	Fleeting episode of monocular, total or partial loss of vision, lasting from a few seconds to a few minutes. May be described as a grey or black curtain coming across the vision.	Refer to GP as per TIA guidance.	Will need screening for cardiovascular risk factors. Standard GP referral letter for TIA as above.

Eye Emergencies: The practitioner's guide

Temporal arteritis/Giant cell arteritis (GCA)	Systemic vasculopathy (disorder of large vessels) e.g. aorta, carotid or temporal artery. Complex, recurring headache.	Main presentation being sudden headache (different to patient's typical headache), generally unilaterally. Over 50s, tenderness to temporal area. Jaw claudication, scalp tenderness. Decreased or loss of vision. Raised ESR.	With ocular symptoms within last 14/7 see Eye A&E same day, request Dr sign form for bloods to include ESR and CRP. If typical symptoms with no eye symptoms, refer to Rheumatology via GP. If non-typical symptoms, without eye symptoms, discuss with Rheumatology. May have local Temporal Arteritis Protocol.	Worth checking history of systemic symptoms over last 1–2/12 (i.e. may have recent history of neck pain and/or headache, weight-loss, malaise/fatigue).
Migraine	Complex, recurring headache.	Classic presentation is unilateral head pain preceded by other sensory symptoms. However there can be bilateral head pain. Headache may last 4–72 hours. Sensory changes include: aura (i.e. scotoma, homonymous hemianopic field defect, tunnel vision or even complete visual loss) developing over 5–20 minutes and resolved within 60 minutes. Scintillating scotoma (area of vision that shimmers, zig zags or glitters) generally starts centrally and expands out before breaking up and disappearing. They may have flashing lights or fractured vision. Photophobia may or may not be a feature. Rarely ptosis. Nausea and vomiting often occur after visual disturbance. Patient may have other sensory auras following the visual disturbance resulting in numbness which may spread over 15–20 minutes and can affect the hands, arms, face and lips. This is slower than the spread with TIA**. Generally under 40s. However TIA should be considered in over 45s.	Suggest analgesia and rest. See GP for future management. If suspect TIA then patient to seek urgent medical review as per guidance for TIA.**	**Standard GP referral letter for TIA.

Visual obscurations		Associated with papilloedema and raised intracranial pressure (ICP).	See Eye A&E.
BRAIN TUMOUR RED FLAGS		According to the NICE guidelines: in spite of the variety of brain tumour pathologies, presentation tends to be related to: ● Headache with cognitive or behavioural symptoms ● Epilepsy ● Progressive focal neurological deficits or ● Headache with raised intracranial pressure. NB. Papilloedema does not necessarily cause altered vision but needs review. In addition be mindful to note when patients present with headache: ● New or altered pattern of headache (i.e. frequency/severity) ● New headaches in over 50s or under 10s ● Headache which wakes patient/morning headaches – raised intracranial pressure causes headaches and also presents as papilloedema ● Headache in patient with cancer, neurofibromatosis or immunodeficiency ● Thunderclap headache (rapid onset) ● Cluster headache.	*Headache without visual disturbance need to see GP unless optometrist referring with papilloedema See Eye A&E if visual disturbance ← To see GP	Focal neurology: ● Lack of co-ordination ● Confusion ● Field defect – occasionally only unilateral field loss ● III nerve defect i.e. ptosis, miosed pupil, downward abducted eye ('down & out') ● Diplopia.

Chapter 3
Differential diagnosis of emergency eye conditions

The practitioner needs to bear in mind that there are six principal ophthalmic emergencies that should be diagnosed and given any preliminary treatment necessary prior to immediate referral to the ophthalmologist, day or night. These are: chemical injury, penetrating injury, acute glaucoma, sudden loss of vision, ophthalmia neonatorum (occasionally), and orbital cellulitis. The following text describes these in some detail and includes a number of less serious presentations that the practitioner needs to know about in order to reach a differential diagnosis and evaluate the urgency of the condition.

Advice is given regarding the speed with which the patient may need to be referred to hospital and some details as to how the patient may be treated are given to facilitate practitioners working in minor injuries units and ophthalmic units. For practitioners working in remote, possibly offshore, settings, this information may prove invaluable as medical evacuation may be delayed. Ophthalmic advice can generally be sought via telephone or radio and it would be prudent to assess the patient thoroughly, carry out any relevant initial treatment and check drug stocks prior to calling.

Always document everything thoroughly to ensure a good referral and avoid unnecessary replication and efforts. Remember that your notes may be required by the police in the event of an injury and may even be required for litigation. Finally, if there is a patient complaint against you, excellent treatment supported by good, legible, unambiguous notes will assist your memory concerning what happened and make a major contribution to your defence.

Chemical injuries

Chemical injuries

Alkali burns to the eye are considered to be potentially the most severe chemical injury, as alkalis are absorbed more rapidly into the tissues of the eye itself (Dua *et al.* 2001), continuing to damage the eye for many hours after the original injury. However, concentrated acids may cause extremely severe damage on immediate contact with the eye structures. This is why serious chemical burns are amongst the most urgent of ophthalmic emergencies.

Alkalis, particularly the lime found in building materials such as cement, plaster and artex, may cause permanent scarring of the cornea, and such chemicals cause many accidents. Due to the frequency and quantities of alkali used, 20% of all occupational eye injuries occur in the construction industry (Welch *et al.* 2001). Equally worrying is the fact that many domestic cleaning solutions are strongly alkali, particularly oven cleaning solutions. Indeed, MacEwan (1999) states that the home is the most common site for a severe eye injury leading to hospital admission.

Speedy irrigation will improve the patient's prognosis. Tap water may be used domestically but sterile normal saline is used in clinical practice, as water is hypotonic to the corneal stroma (Kuckelkorn *et al.* 2002).

If the patient, or their companion, rings for advice, clearly state that the eye must be immediately washed out with plenty of water. First-aid irrigation should last at least ten minutes. Suggest ways in which to do this.

- The patient may hold their head under a gently flowing tap, or shower.
- A wash basin can be filled with water and the patient can open their eye under the water.
- An egg cup can be used quickly as an eye bath.
- Children can be wrapped in a blanket or large towel, and the eye irrigated using a small jug or other suitable small, clean container.
- Industrial eye wash bottles are helpful as an emergency quick wash but further liberal washing is always needed. An eye wash bottle may be used by the patient during a long car transfer to the hospital or treatment centre.

On receiving the telephone call, alert other staff to the patient's expected arrival and prepare the equipment required to irrigate the patient's eye(s) thoroughly. If the patient has a severe chemical injury, perhaps even involving both eyes, a litre bag of normal saline and an IV-giving set may be prepared for initial irrigation.

Figure 3.1

Severe chemical injury

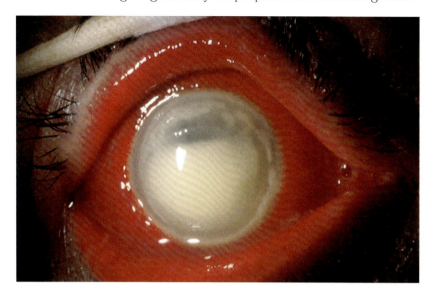

Immediate action

On arrival in the department or surgery, if you have the test paper required, the pH of both the patient's eyes should be tested (see 'Checking the pH' in Chapter 9). A pH of 7 to 7.5 is considered normal. Above this level, the patient has been in contact with an alkali; below this level, the patient has an acid injury.

Always test the pH of both eyes. Sometimes both are affected, even when the patient thinks that the chemical only went into one eye. It is also useful as a comparison if only one eye is affected, as the pH may vary slightly from person to person.

The patient's eye(s) should be irrigated until the pH returns to normal (see 'Irrigating an eye' in Chapter 9) or until the ophthalmologist gives permission to stop. Instil a local anaesthetic eyedrop such as oxybuprocaine hydrochloride prior to washing and at intervals during the procedure as the irrigating fluid will also rapidly leech out the anaesthetic drops.

Always check for lumps of cement or artex in the corners of the eyes and under the eyelids, ensuring the eyelids are everted to check the tarsal plate. Remove any debris promptly with cotton wool buds (this is referred to as fornix sweeping). If the debris is difficult to remove, try an 'arrow head' swab or a fine pair of forceps such as Mathalone forceps.

When the eye(s) have been washed for a sufficient length of time, perhaps for about ten minutes for a minor injury but at least 30 minutes for a major injury, check the pH again. About ten minutes should be allowed to elapse before doing so, in order that it is not just the irrigation fluid that has just been poured around the eye that is being tested.

With an alkali injury, it is not so much the quantity of fluid that is being used, as the time which is taken bathing the eye with a slow stream of neutral fluid to leech out the alkali, which is important.

Between irrigation sessions, check the visual acuity. The history, which should have been gathered during the irrigation procedure, can be written up.

Morgan lens

A Morgan lens can be used to irrigate the eye(s) whilst staff attend to the patient's other injuries. They are reasonably expensive. However, the device can save practitioner time in a busy ED department, but should only be used after documented lid eversion and fornix sweeping (Chan *et al*. 2005). The manufacturers of the Morgan lens recommend use of Ringer's Lactate solution for irrigation, stating that it is closer to the pH of human tears. They refer to unpublished and unreferenced research performed for them to indicate that irrigation of the eyes with Ringer's Lactate solution and the Morgan lens is 'more comfortable to patients' (www.morganlens.com/faq.html).

Documentation

Documentation must include:
- time of injury
- substance to which the patient has been exposed
- duration of the exposure until the irrigation was started
- pH on arrival (and time of testing)
- duration of the irrigation – how much fluid used
- eyelid eversion
- fornix sweeping
- pH following irrigation (and time of testing).

If the pH has not returned to normal, reassure the patient and commence washing again, for at least 20 minutes, document and reassess.

Differential diagnosis of emergency eye conditions

 Major chemical injuries

Symptoms of major chemical injuries:
- visual acuity may be affected
- difficulty in getting the pH of the eye back to normal
- limbal ischaemia (seen as white, avascular areas at the corneal margins on an eye which is otherwise red)
- avascular areas on eyelid eversion
- severe corneal staining
- hazy cornea.

Management

Patients with major injuries should be referred to the ophthalmologist immediately following initial irrigation. You will need to relay the specific information you have recorded and the results of your eye examination. Arrange for continuing cycles of irrigation whilst the patient waits. They may require hospital admission for specialised treatment. This is likely to include vitamin C eye drops (Brodovsky *et al.* 2000), intensive steroid eye drops and topical antibiotics. Oral prescriptions may include vitamin C tablets. Ensure that the patient is also prescribed oral analgesia.

Minor chemical injuries

Minor injuries, for example perfume and dilute shampoo in the eye, may be treated by an experienced practitioner, provided that:
- the pH of the eye is normal
- the vision in the affected eye is satisfactory
- any corneal staining is minimal
- a check has been made under the eyelids for avascular areas
- there is no limbal ischaemia.

Management

If you have not referred the patient to the ophthalmologist as an emergency, remember that all patients with chemical injuries will require chloramphenicol ointment or fusidic acid 1% (Fucithalmic) after treatment for three to five days after trauma (Fraser *et al.* 2001). This is because irrigation and handling of the eyelashes and lids may cause infection to be introduced, particularly as the normal, protective tear film is washed away. Additionally, the patient may develop a sore, red eye following the exposure to the chemical. The eye will be dry, having had the normal tear film very effectively washed away, and ointment is a comforting means of providing the antibiotic cover required.

Advise that, although sore at first, the eye symptoms will slowly clear. The patient should telephone for advice immediately if symptoms worsen. By the day after the injury, the patient will be beginning to feel much better.

CS spray (tear gas)

(This is not normally considered an emergency, but included here with chemical injuries for the sake of completeness.)

CS is a chlorine-based spray that reacts with moisture in the eyes, nose and throat to produce hydrochloric acid. Spray canisters are used by the police to control riots or individual violence.

Practitioners should wear gloves when handling these patients, treat any breathing difficulties first and then make sure that the patient's contact lenses, if worn, are removed.

There has been no hard evidence of harmful long-term effects or deaths from CS spray (DH 1999). However, CS is an irritant and can cause the following general symptoms:

- irritation of the skin, eyes and mucous membranes, temporary loss of co-ordination, watering eyes, running nose
- ocular symptoms such as conjunctival redness, pain in the eyes, reduced visual acuity, lacrimation, blepharospasm, photophobia, skin erythema and eyelid erythema.

Treatment

- Expose the patient to plenty of fresh air, for example by sitting them by an open door or window. You may direct a fan on the patient, situated to blow residual gas out of the room.
- Wear gloves when handling or examining the eye to prevent self-contamination.
- Irrigate with sterile water or saline to get rid of any other foreign bodies which may have entered the eye after fan treatment.
- Reassure the patient that the effects are not long-term. Ask them not to rub their face, as this may re-activate the irritant.
- Check visual acuity and examine the eye thoroughly, using fluorescein, to check that the patient's eye symptoms do not have any other cause.
- Treat any thermal burns or contact dermatitis that may be present, according to local protocols.

Pepper spray (oleoresin capsicum)

Pepper spray contains a similar chemical to that occurring in naturally growing peppers. It is known to be biodegradable and doesn't linger in clothing or the areas in which it was sprayed. For these reasons, it doesn't require any special decontamination procedures.

Pepper spray is used to cause temporary blindness and its effects are tearing, blepharospasm, redness and burning of the skin. It may cause upper respiratory tract problems and temporary blindness. Bates (2004) notes that the effects normally last only 15 to 30 minutes. Research by Vesaluoma *et al.* (2000) found that, when used according to the manufacturer's recommendations, pepper spray caused occasional areas of epithelial cell damage that healed within a day and some changes in corneal sensitivity lasting up to a week.

Treatment

- Wear gloves to deal with the patient to prevent self-contamination.
- If the patient is wearing contact lenses, remove them as soon as possible.
- Irrigate the eyes as for any other chemical injury.
- Wash the face with cold water, as the skin pores will remain closed, and the pepper won't penetrate deeper into the skin.
- Do not use anything oily on the skin as this will tend to trap the pepper on the skin.
- When supplying an antibiotic to prevent chemical conjunctivitis, choose eye drops if possible.

As with CS spray, it is not normally necessary for patients exposed to pepper sprays to require hospital treatment, given that the effects are normally, as Bates (2004) states, short-lived and self-limiting, unless the spray has not been used in accordance with the manufacturer's guidelines. If there is no clear history of exposure to either CS gas or pepper spray, check the pH of the eyes, just in case another chemical is implicated and check under the eyelids for foreign bodies.

Paint in the eye

Paint will cause stinging and irritation to the eyes. Particularly unpleasant paints are 'anti-graffiti' paints, which contain naphtha, and other solvent-borne synthetic paints. These should be treated in the same way as chemical injuries (above). Excess paint can be satisfactorily removed from the eyelids and face using liquid paraffin.

Major eye injuries

Major eye injuries

Emergency eye injuries are responsible for 50% of attendances at Eye ED departments in the UK (Vernon 1999). Many of these injuries are fairly trivial, but it is important that the practitioner does not miss a potentially serious eye injury in the otherwise well person.

The two major types of injury are:

blunt injuries – from objects small enough to fit inside the orbital rim (shuttlecocks, squash balls, champagne corks, golf balls and knuckles). The sudden rise in pressure within the orbit and distortion of the eye may cause severe damage and possible rupture of the eye. In the 1980s sports-associated eye injuries became responsible for most cases of hospitalised eye trauma (MacEwan 1999) but trends are changing due to increased use of protective eye wear.

penetrating injuries – from microscopic tears, caused, for example, by the point of a dart, abrasion from a thorn bush through to massive, complex lacerations, for example from a shattered grinding wheel or some other large metallic object flying off a moving machine. Penetrating injuries following road accidents have declined as a result of seat belt legislation but eye trauma following air bag inflation is a possibility. Some of the above injuries may also involve orbital fractures.

Figure 3.2

Penetrating injury

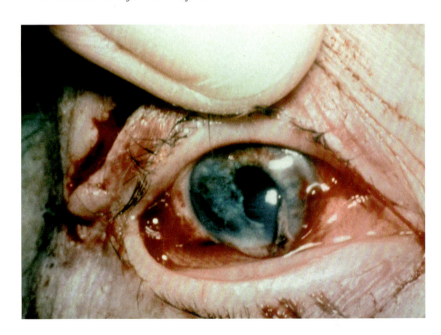

Differential diagnosis of emergency eye conditions

Be alert for the possibility of small intra-ocular foreign bodies. The history of an injury is of critical importance in suggesting possible penetration of the eye by a foreign body which might otherwise be overlooked. A person using a hammer and chisel without eye protection is at particular risk, as are people using grinding wheels without eye protection or someone who has been near an explosion of any kind.

Always get an ophthalmic opinion if the history of the injury mentions being near to any kind of explosion, hammering (most especially metal on metal), broken glass or broken spectacles. Be aware that initially undetected retained intra-ocular foreign bodies may give rise to severe orbital complications (Fulcher *et al.* 2002).

A comprehensive, competent assessment and examination will avoid potential litigation problems. History-taking should therefore be careful and accurate and include exactly what the patient was doing around the time of the injury, and whether eye protection was being worn.

Signs

- If a sharp object was involved, tissue from the iris, choroid or retina may be seen plugging a corneal or scleral wound.

- An irregular pupil.

Be cautious. Something as apparently benign as a subconjunctival haemorrhage following trauma may conceal an underlying penetration, especially if the haemorrhage has a bullous appearance.

Examination

Visual acuity
Visual acuity may be reduced in comparison to the other eye, especially if the injury is severe and has involved the lens of the eye.

However, if there has been only a tiny penetration, visual acuity may be normal.

The eyelids
Examine the skin around the orbit and eyelids for possible penetrating wounds but avoid pressure on the eye itself during examination.

Acute swelling may make examination extremely difficult. An assistant may be required to help retract swollen eyelids and dry gauze swabs placed over the upper and lower eyelids may be used to provide some grip on the swollen skin prior to retraction.

The conjunctiva

- Look very carefully for any clues suggesting penetration, such as a bulging subconjunctival haemorrhage.
- Look for any possibility that the iris, choroid or retina is appearing subconjunctivally.

The cornea

- Look for any evidence of a full thickness laceration, looking especially for an iris prolapse plugging a wound of either the cornea or sclera. Remember that a tiny cut may heal within hours, so it is important to develop slit lamp skills that enable you to examine the full thickness of the cornea.
- Use and document the results of Seidel's test to check for a leaking cornea (see 'Seidel test to detect a wound leak' in Chapter 9) but bear in mind that a negative result does not necessarily mean that there has not been a corneal penetration. Only a positive Seidel's test is significant.

The pupil

- Look for any abnormality, especially an irregular, 'teardrop' shape.
- Check pupil reactions of both eyes. There may be a traumatic mydriasis, or an RAPD (see 'Checking for relative afferent pupillary defect' in Chapter 9).

Eye movements

Restricted eye movement manifest as a reduction in the upward gaze of the affected eye may indicate a 'blow out' fracture of the orbital floor (see 'Checking eye movements' in Chapter 9).

Intra-ocular pressure

In a person with a suspicious history but no clear evidence of a penetration or intra-ocular foreign body, the intra-ocular pressure may be measured very carefully using a Goldman applanation tonometer. A lower pressure in the affected eye may deepen a suspicion that there has been a penetration, but normal intra-ocular pressure does not necessarily mean that there has not been a penetration. Only a positive result is significant.

Management of severe injuries

Diagnosis may be obvious within minutes of the patient being examined by the practitioner with a pen torch. Document a thorough history and examination and then seek an immediate ophthalmic opinion.

Whether or not you attempt to measure visual acuity is a matter of judgement based on the general condition of the patient and the severity of the eye condition.

Diagnostic tests that may be ordered by the ophthalmologist to check for known or possible intra-ocular foreign bodies include:

- plain X-ray films to detect the number and location of radio opaque foreign bodies
- ultrasound to detect radio opaque foreign bodies in the anterior orbit
- a computer tomogram (CT) scan to detect most radio opaque foreign bodies, including stone, aluminium, lead-free glass, copper and steel
- a magnetic resonance imaging (MRI) scan may be used to detect vegetable and wooden foreign bodies.

Once a diagnosis of penetrating injury or intra-ocular foreign body has been made, an emergency admission will be arranged and the ophthalmologist will remove the foreign body or attempt to repair the eye as soon as possible because of the risk of severe infection developing within the eye. Given the complex and increasingly sophisticated nature of the surgery, a fully staffed ophthalmic theatre in the daytime is often preferred.

IV antibiotics are normally given for at least 24 hours following major eye trauma, followed by oral antibiotics. Eye drop treatments are likely to include antibiotics, mydriatics and steroids. It may be days or weeks following the original injury before the ophthalmologist is able to say whether or not the eye has been 'saved'.

Acute glaucoma

Acute glaucoma

This condition occurs in hypermetropic (long-sighted) people, with shallow anterior chambers (Kotecha 2002). The condition affects more women than men, in the ratio four to one (Kaiser *et al.* 2004). There are two reasons for this – women comprise a larger proportion of the older population and may have slightly smaller eyes, with shallower anterior chambers, than men.

Typically the patient presents with a history of sudden severe eye pain, often accompanied by nausea. The visual acuity is grossly reduced, often to as low as 6/60 or even 'count fingers'. Immediate treatment is required to prevent permanent visual damage.

Causes of acute (closed angle) glaucoma

Tumosa (2003) identifies the major causative factor as being an anatomically shallow anterior chamber, particularly at the periphery. The risk of developing acute glaucoma builds up throughout life as the lens continues to grow, pushing the iris forward. Eventually the peripheral margin of the iris presses against the lens, inhibiting the flow of aqueous into the anterior chamber. Tumosa describes the mechanism whereby aqueous fluid builds up in the posterior chamber, pushing the middle of the iris forward, effectively sealing the drainage access to the trabecular meshwork.

This mechanical problem is not confined to the very elderly, and 1:1000 people over age 40 are said to be at risk of this condition (Dayan 1996). Most long-sighted people, however, retain adequate drainage and never develop acute glaucoma.

'Warning' attacks

Your patient may already have suffered from less severe, 'warning' attacks, which typically occur in the evening, when lighting is subdued and the pupils tend naturally to dilate. When this happens, the person may notice the onset of severe frontal headache, blurred vision and haloes (rainbow-coloured rings around lights, caused by corneal oedema). These warning attacks tend to clear by morning. This is because the pupil tends to constrict spontaneously during sleep and the pressure returns to normal, known as 'sleep-induced miosis' (Skuta 1994). If you suspect this is happening to a patient in your care, you should arrange for an urgent ophthalmic clinic referral.

Eventually the patient has an attack of raised intra-ocular pressure which does not clear spontaneously. This will happen over time or it may be brought on more quickly for the following reasons:

- The use of a mydriatic (dilating) eye drop, or antimuscinaric drugs (antipsychotic drugs, antihistamines, anti-emetics or atropine, for example, in connection with general anaesthetic) precipitates a severe attack. Check the patient's recent drug history.
- Going out in the dark or visiting the cinema, causing prolonged pupil dilation.
- Overwork, anxiety and personal stress are all said to be contributory factors. The mechanism is uncertain and unproved but it may be that chronic stressors act on the sympathetic nervous system to produce pupil dilation.
- Alcohol may bring on acute glaucoma, insofar as the effects of drinking a large volume of fluid will temporarily raise the circulating volume and possibly raise the intra-ocular pressure.

Signs

- Shallow anterior chamber
- A crimson red eye with a crimson flush round the cornea
- Hazy cornea – the raised pressure inside the eye has forced excess fluid into the cornea
- Fixed, semi-dilated pupil which may appear slightly oval
- Discoloured iris to brown/green – the raised pressure is causing iris ischaemia
- Engorged iris vessels (if you can obtain a view of the iris)

Symptoms

- Sudden onset (often within 30 to 60 minutes) of severe one-sided eye pain, concentrated in the brow or orbit or present as a generalised brow or headache (Duane and Jaegar 1992)

- Vomiting or prostration
- Rapid drop in visual acuity of the affected eye – haloes around lights, blurred vision

Diagnosis

Check the history, make a pen torch examination and try gentle finger palpation of both eyes. The affected eye will feel very hard to the touch.

Figure 3.3

Acute glaucoma

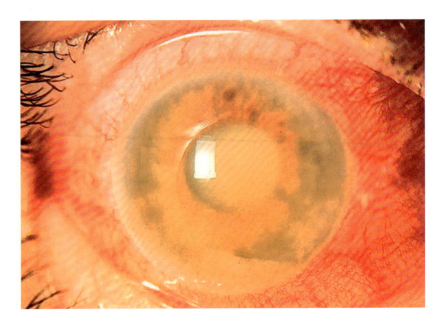

Ophthalmologists will not commit themselves to a precise time but there is generally thought to be about 24 hours from the onset of this condition in which to provide treatment before the patient suffers irreversible visual loss in the affected eye. Older patients in particular often delay seeking help until they are quite ill, so immediate referral is essential. Both eyes will need to be treated promptly as the other eye is at risk of developing the same condition.

Slit lamp examination will include an intra ocular pressure (IOP) check, using the Goldman applanation tonometer. The IOP may be raised as high as 50 to 70 mm Hg. The cornea is very oedematous and fragile so be careful not to cause an accidental abrasion while making your measurement. The view of the anterior chamber will be hazy.

Ring the ophthalmologist for an immediate referral.

Confusing presentations

Very occasionally a patient may not complain explicitly of eye pain, but present instead with malaise, abdominal pain and possibly headache (Galloway *et al.* 2002 and Gandhewa and Kamath 2005). Such patients have occasionally been misdiagnosed with gastro-enteritis and valuable treatment time lost. The quality of physical examination, particularly of the red eye, which will be present, should prevent mistakes occurring. As Dayan

Differential diagnosis of emergency eye conditions

(1996) points out, acutely ill elderly people may not volunteer specific eye symptoms.

Hospital treatment

Hospital treatment is focused on reduction of intra-ocular pressure. Local treatment protocols vary and may include the following

- 500 mg acetazolamide (Diamox) stat IV.
- 250 mg acetazolamide tabs QDS. (Remember to consider the injection in calculating how much acetazolamide has been given on the first day. 1g is the total recommended dose in 24 hours. Very occasionally this is exceeded on ophthalmic consultant instruction only.)
- Pilocarpine hydrochloride 4% is instilled to miose the pupil of the affected eye and to pull the drainage angle open once the intra-ocular pressure has fallen to about 40 mm Hg. Pilocarpine is thought to be relatively ineffective whilst the pressure is very high, as the circulation to the ciliary body and iris is reduced and the drug is not readily absorbed. The ophthalmologist will advise regarding frequency of dosage.
- Pilocarpine hydrochloride 2% to miose the pupil of the unaffected eye and prevent an attack occurring in the second eye.
- Apraclonidine hydrochloride (Iopidine) to decrease the production of aqueous humour.

Osmotic diuretics

- Rarely, persistent raised intra-ocular pressure (IOP) may require the use of IV Mannitol infusion to create a forced diuresis and temporarily lower the IOP.
- Oral glycerin (Glycerol) is rarely used these days.

Laser

- Yttrium Aluminium Garnet (YAG) laser iridotomy to create an additional route for aqueous to circulate into the drainage angle once the pressure has reduced, the cornea is clear and the patient is comfortable. Generally the unaffected eye is treated with YAG laser also to prevent similar problems.

Surgery

- Iridectomy – this has been almost entirely replaced by laser treatment.

In remote locations, discuss with the ophthalmologist immediately via telephone or radio. Anti-emetics and analgesia will be required in addition to the eye drops above. If transfer to acute services is liable to be delayed, and you have access to controlled drugs, ask the ophthalmologist whether the muscarinic drugs morphine, heroin and pethidine, which also promote pupil miosis (Fedder *et al.* 1984), might be indicated for analgesia.

Other causes of an acute rise in intra-ocular pressure

Rubeosis iridis

Rubeosis iridis (neovascularisation of the iris) is a proliferation of abnormal blood vessels growing across the iris (hence the name rubeosis) due to retinal ischaemia, possibly from advanced diabetic retinopathy or central retinal vein occlusion. The new blood vessels can occlude the drainage angle which causes a rise in the intra-ocular pressure.

Figure 3.4

Neovascular (rubeotic) glaucoma

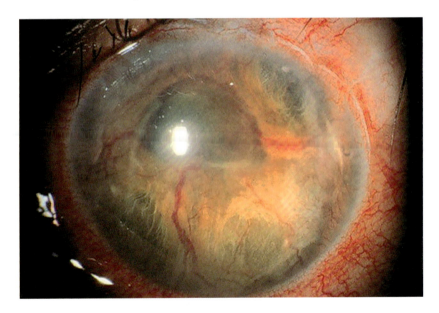

This condition may also be called thrombotic glaucoma if it follows a central retinal vein occlusion (CRVO) or branch vein occlusion (BRVO) as patients are likely to develop this condition some weeks after the original sight loss, hence being sometimes called 'hundred day glaucoma'. This should not occur in British society, either for people with diabetic eye disease or vein occlusions, as they will normally have follow-up clinic appointments and preventive laser treatment. The symptoms of this type of glaucoma are like those of acute glaucoma – pain, red eye.

Refer to ophthalmologist.

Overnight, ring the ophthalmologist for advice. This is not an emergency in terms of being able to save vision because it has already been lost. The emergency is the management of the patient's acute pain and the nausea which is likely to accompany it.

Hyphaema

Blood in the anterior chamber may block the drainage of aqueous. The patient with hyphaema may also have reduced vision, pain, nausea and a hazy cornea.

Ring the ophthalmologist.

Post-intra-ocular surgery

Surgical debris or resulting inflammation may block the drainage angle. Silicone oil from retinal surgery may result in pressure rise.

Ring the ophthalmologist.

Inflammation

Raised intra-ocular pressure may result from anterior uveitis as a complication of herpes zoster ophthalmicus.

Ring the ophthalmologist.

Swollen lens

A swollen lens may be taking up more space at the front of the eye and be blocking the drainage angle. This may happen after the initial repair of a penetrating eye injury or because an untreated age-related cataract has become hypermature.

Ring the ophthalmologist.

Ophthalmia neonatorum

Ophthalmia neonatorum

This is a very severe purulent conjunctivitis, appearing in a baby in the first 21 days of life, and is a notifiable disease under the Public Health Infectious Diseases Regulation Act 1988 (Public Health England and Wales 1988). It is acquired during the vaginal birth process and may be caused in various ways.

Differential diagnosis

Physical immaturity

Some babies have naturally slightly sticky eyes in the first few months following birth, due to immaturity of the tear passages. Advise the mother to clean round the eyes with cotton wool moistened in cool, boiled water regularly. Antibiotics are rarely necessary for this problem. If it does not clear during the first few months of life, refer to the ophthalmic OPD clinic.

Most of these sticky eyes clear gradually and spontaneously when the tear passages gradually canalise as the child nears their first birthday.

Gonococcus

Vernon (1999) suggests that if the infection manifests itself in the first few days of life, it is likely to be gonococcal. The baby with a gonococcal infection may have swollen eyelids and very purulent sticky eyes. Open the baby's eyes gently to take a look. The baby has very strong muscles surrounding the eyes, and will squeeze strongly to resist you, and it's not unusual for the eyelids to evert spontaneously as you pull them open. Pus may squirt out from under the eyelids if the infection is severe, so be careful. You may also see red, bleeding conjunctiva lining the eyelids, with pseudomembranes, composed of congealing purulent material. Refer a presentation of this severity to the ophthalmologist or paediatrician urgently, particularly if you note any corneal epithelial loss.

Once a gonococcal infection gets established, there is the possibility of the baby's delicate corneas perforating spontaneously if urgent treatment with the right antibiotics is not administered. If only one eye is infected, advise the mother to lie the baby in the cot with the infected eye nearest to the mattress, so that any discharge is less likely to infect the other eye.

Chlamydia

If the eye infection manifests itself on or after about day five, it is likely to be a chlamydia infection (Vernon 1999). The baby needs to be seen by a paediatrician, as the condition also produces systemic symptoms and effects and needs to be treated with systemic erythromycin.

Herpes simplex

In late pregnancy the risk of neonatal transmission is greatest, occurring in about 40% of cases (NICE 2012).

Bacterial conjunctivitis

It is possible that the baby may have contracted the eye infection from another member of the family with conjunctivitis.

Hospital treatment

Hospital treatment for ophthalmia neonatorum is likely to include:

- immediate swabs and slides for gram stain and sensitivities (Do not instil fluorescein until swabs have been taken for chlamydial studies.)
- oral antibiotics and hourly eye drops, for which mother and baby may be admitted.

Remember that both parents will need psychological support and will require checks and treatment for sexually transmitted disease once a definite diagnosis of the baby's condition has been reached.

Remember to check for any obvious trauma to the conjunctiva and cornea that may have occurred during the birth process or any tiny scratch that the baby may have caused to his or her own cornea.

Orbital infections

Orbital infections

These infections affect people of all ages. There are two types.

Preseptal cellulitis

Preseptal cellulitis is often seen in children. It may result from infection from a stye, infected cyst or insect bite. The child presents with a swollen, painful eyelid but is otherwise well, with a normal temperature. Oral antibiotics are usually prescribed for children with this infection, as it can lead to orbital cellulitis. Ear, Nose and Throat referral may be required. Unless there is an obvious eye-related cause, this problem may be linked to a sinus infection.

The key difference between this condition and orbital cellulitis is that this problem lies in front of the orbital septum – a fibrous layer of tissue attached at the orbital margin and lining both eyelids, effectively separating the preseptal space from the orbital contents.

Eye Emergencies: The practitioner's guide

Figure 3.5
Preseptal cellulitis

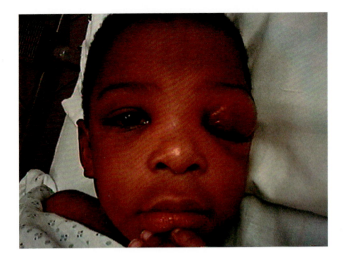

All patients with preseptal cellulitis should be followed up regularly to ensure reduction in swelling and general improvement with the antibiotic treatment as it could lead to orbital cellulitis. Guideline for first follow-up interval would be after 48 hours, to allow the antibiotic to take effect, unless, of course, further symptoms develop.

Orbital cellulitis

Orbital cellulitis is less common and is an infection of the soft tissues lying within the orbit. 60% of these infections arise from the sinuses – mainly the ethmoid sinus (Lafferty 2014). Other causes may be from infected superficial injuries and injuries of the skin around the orbit; infections of the throat or middle ear, following eye surgery; or blood-borne infections from remote septic foci (rare, but possible).

Orbital cellulitis is potentially life-threatening, as it can spread to the venous drainage system of the orbit to the cavernous sinus in the brain (containing arteries and nerves) causing meningitis, intracranial infection, septicemia and death.

You should safely recognise this infection as it is characterised by:

 Symptoms
- Patient feeling and looking generally unwell
- Severe orbital pain
- Raised temperature (very rarely, this may not be so)
- Possible reduced vision

Signs

Initially:

- eyelid swelling and redness
- conjunctivitis
- chemosis (conjunctival swelling)

Later:

- ptosis (upper eyelid drooping)
- proptosis (protrusion of the eye on the affected side)
- double vision (due to the proptosis)
- diminished colour vision
- an afferent pupil defect.

In this condition, these are very serious symptoms indeed.

Figure 3.6

Orbital cellulitis (note the conjunctival chemosis)

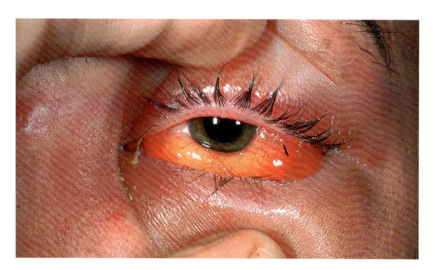

Management

Refer now! Treatment is likely to include:

- emergency admission
- cephalosporins, e.g. cefuroxime plus metronidazole
- for people allergic to penicillin, clindamycin plus a quinolone such as ciprofloxacin.

Most general hospitals now have specific guidelines on the management of sepsis and require intravenous antibiotics to be given within one hour of the patient's presentation. The UK Sepsis Trust lays out clear guidelines for assessing patients with suspected infection and advises that sepsis screening should be linked to NEWS (National Early Warning Score) (UK Sepsis Trust 2014).

Sudden painless loss of vision

Sudden loss of vision may occur at different stages in the life span, and result from a variety of causes. It is treated as an emergency if the loss has just happened or occurred within the week. Your level of ophthalmic knowledge may not be sufficient for you to distinguish between the many types of loss of vision described below but the information given will help you in doing a preliminary 'work up'. Some guidance is given regarding the possible urgency of referral, but if you are in a quandary, always ring the ophthalmologist for advice.

General history

General history should include the following:

- age
- time of day the problem occurred
- whether the visual loss is transient or constant
- how the patient noticed the problem and whether it could have existed for some time, but have just been noticed
- whether one eye or both is affected
- whether there a history of injury, e.g. a recent fall
- any previous, fleeting losses of vision
- general health of the patient – check history for diabetes, cerebrovascular disease, hypertension and atrial fibrillation
- whether the patient is a smoker and/or heavy drinker.

Examination

Examination should include the following:

- testing visual acuity accurately
- checking eye movements (see 'Checking eye movements' in Chapter 9)
- checking for presence or absence of a pupillary defect (see 'Checking for relative afferent pupillary defect' in Chapter 9)

and also, if possible:

- examination of the anterior chamber of the eye on the slit lamp
- checking of the intra-ocular pressure.

People aged between 50 and 70 are statistically the most vulnerable to conditions which affect circulation at the back of the eye, with the highest incidence in men (Hammond 2000). Possible causes include the following.

Differential diagnosis of emergency eye conditions

Amaurosis fugax

Amaurosis fugax affects one eye, causing sudden painless partial or total loss of vision which lasts from a few seconds to about 20 minutes. It is a significant indication of systemic disease, being caused by an embolus which has resulted in a sudden temporary blockage to the arterial circulation of the retina. (It can also be one of the features of a transient ischaemic attack.)

Generally, this is an older patient, possibly with an existing history of diabetes and or circulatory problems. Younger patients may have a history of heart valve disease, drug abuse or a blood-clotting disorder, for example sickle cell disease.

Symptoms

- A grey or black 'curtain', rapidly closing off vision from above or one side
- A history of more generalised transient ischaemic attacks

Management

- Diagnosis is on history alone.
- Check pulse for regularity, blood pressure, heart sounds and whether you can detect a carotid bruit.
- Make a telephone referral to the cardiologists within 24 hours.
- Have an urgent telephone discussion with the ophthalmologist (not in the middle of the night), as differental diagnosis includes temporal arteritis, papilloedema, optic neuritis and raised intra-ocular pressure.
- Arrange blood tests for erythrocyte sedimentation rate (ESR), full blood count (FBC), glucose and lipids.
- Commence aspirin 75 mg daily (if not contra-indicated).
- If the patient is a smoker, advise them to stop smoking.

Differential diagnosis

If the reported transient loss of vision affects both eyes, the patient may have suffered a vertebrobasilar transient ischaemic attack (TIA) caused by stenosis in either the vertebral or basilar arteries, affecting the occipital cortical circulation bilaterally. If the patient had simultaneous vertigo, this is likely to be the case. Refer to the physicians.

Chronic papilloedema is also likely to be bilateral. It may cause loss of peripheral vision and transient general loss, so check the optic discs and refer to the physicians.

Amaurosis fugax is also an important symptom which precedes permanent visual loss in 44% of patients with temporal arteritis (Salvarini *et al.* 2002). Refer to the physicians if you suspect this.

Central retinal artery occlusion (CRAO)

Patients complaining of sudden painless loss of vision occurring within the past hour may have an arterial occlusion. This is usually caused by an embolus (of fibrin and platelets or cholesterol or calcium) from the carotid artery or from the heart.

Typically, the patient may be between 50 and 80 years old and have other systemic health problems, diagnosed or undiagnosed, such as hypertension, hyperlipidaemia, diabetes, circulatory problems such as atrial fibrillation. Krishnan *et al.* (2004) state that retinal artery occlusion is a marker for significant carotid artery and heart disease.

Symptoms

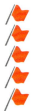

- Very acute loss of vision
- Problem came 'out of the blue'
- Condition is painless and the eye looks 'normal'
- An RAPD (see Chapter 9) on the affected side
- Vision likely to be reduced to count fingers or hand movements.

Firm diagnosis is made by dilating the pupil and ophthalmoscopy, which reveals a partial or complete block in the retinal circulation. The patient is seen to have a pale optic disc, cloudy retina and a

Figure 3.7

Central retinal artery occlusion

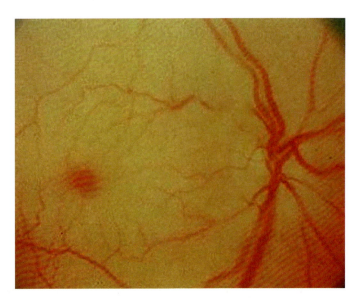

cherry-red spot in the macula. Retinal survival time following the initial infarction has been estimated at 97 minutes by Hayreh *et al.* (2004), hence the urgency of referral, but most ophthalmologists would attempt treatment if the patient presented within 24 hours.

Management

Refer now! Ring the ophthalmologist, day or night, for urgent advice.

The patient requires immediate referral, as these are the symptoms of a potentially life-threatening medical situation for the patient. Aspirin therapy may be commenced by the ophthalmologist.

Treatment

The priorities are to dilate the retinal blood vessels and reduce the intra-ocular pressure below normal levels.

- The patient may be asked to breathe in and out of a paper bag. The purpose of this is to increase the blood CO_2 levels and induce vasodilation.
- Eye massage, for periods of 5 to 15 seconds for about 15 minutes, is undertaken to promote fast drainage of aqueous through the trabecular meshwork, causing reduction of intra-ocular pressure which may result in the embolic material shifting.
- IV acetazolamide (Diamox) and paracentesis of the anterior chamber may be tried in an attempt to further reduce the pressure inside the eye and increase retinal perfusion.
- Fraser *et al.* (2001) suggest that if the patient normally takes glyceryl trinitrate (GTN) for angina, it would do no harm for them to take an extra dose as it might have a beneficial effect on the central retinal artery.

It is important for the patient to know that everything possible is being done to save their sight. However, Fraser and Siriwardena (2002) caution that there is currently no satisfactory evidence to decide which interventions for acute CRAO are effective and it is unwise to over-reassure the patient as the visual prognosis is poor.

There will be an urgent referral to a physician to manage the patient's overall condition.

Branch retinal artery occlusion (BRAO)

This may be defined as a blockage in a branch of the central retinal artery. The causes and symptoms are also similar to those of CRAO, but cause a partial loss of vision, corresponding to the area of retina affected. The treatment is similar but the visual loss is less catastrophic and there may be some visual recovery.

Central retinal vein occlusion (CRVO)

This is caused by a blood clot in the central retinal vein and tends to occur in older people. Diverse underlying factors are cited in the literature, the principal amongst them being hypertension, coronary artery disease, diabetes, hyperlipidaemia, pre-existing glaucoma and ocular hypertension. In younger patients it has been associated with the use of the contraceptive pill and AIDS.

Signs and symptoms

- Visual complaints vary from painless mild to moderate blurring of vision to reduced vision down to 6/60, 6/36 or even hand movements or perception of light of fairly sudden onset, which may be transient.
- There is no pain.
- The eye looks normal.

Diagnosis is reached by dilating the pupil and observing for:

- swollen tortuous retinal veins
- diffuse haemorrhage
- swollen disc, cotton wool spots.

Figure 3.8

Central retinal vein occlusion

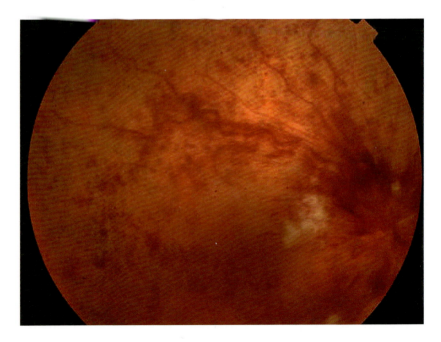

Management

Vision loss is said to be less catastrophic than with central retinal artery occlusion at presentation, but without excellent ophthalmoscope skills you will be unable to distinguish between the two.

- Check for RAPD, blood pressure, blood glucose (or urinalysis) and ESR.
- Ring the ophthalmologist immediately, even at night, as for suspected artery occlusion (unless you have the ophthalmic skills to make a firm diagnosis) and ask for advice.

Treatment

Having confirmed the diagnosis, the ophthalmologist will refer the patient to the physicians. Close ophthalmic follow-up will be required in the weeks following the problem as laser treatment may be indicated to prevent the growth of new vessels in response to the retinal damage, which, without laser treatment to the retina, may result in vitreous haemorrhages or rubeotic damage to the trabecular meshwork. The prognosis for visual recovery was historically poor.

However recent developments have shown an improvement in vision with injectable anti-VEGF agents into the eye, though many trials are still ongoing (Mitry *et al.*, 2013). There is also the possibility of implanting steroid by intravitreal injection such as Ozurdex (dexamethasone 0.7mg) which treats the macular oedema following CRVO and can aid in improving visual outcomes. These treatments would be managed in an ophthalmic department.

Branch vein occlusion

Symptoms are similar to the above, but there will be a visual field defect which relates to the vein affected. It is still possible for the patient to have normal central vision if the macula is not involved. Manage as above.

Visual distortion

Problems with the macula such as oedema and neovascularisation are likely to cause distorted vision. Straight lines, for example around door frames, are described by the patient as being bowed. This may be the first indication of serious macula pathology.

Micropsia, seeing things smaller with one eye, may indicate central serous maculopathy.

Management

Urgent telephone discussion with ophthalmologist (but not during the night). An urgent clinic referral and specialised ophthalmic tests are likely to ensue.

Vitreous haemorrhage

A vitreous haemorrhage is symptomatic of other problems at the back of the eye. It may be associated with diabetic eye disease, retinal tear, vitreous detachment and hypertensive retinopathy.

Symptoms

- Vision may be reduced in the affected eye, depending on the location of the haemorrhage.
- The patient may give a history of a shower of red floaters, or complain of the presence of a new black blob.

Figure 3.9

Vitreous haemorrhage

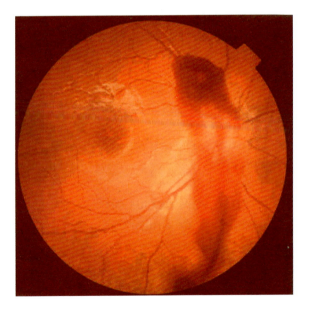

Ask:

- is there a history of trauma?
- is the patient on warfarin or aspirin?
- is the patient diabetic?

Signs

Red reflex on the affected side may be dulled. (A 'red reflex' may be seen on photographs of people with normal eyes following flash photography. To check the red reflex, use a direct ophthalmoscope close to your own eye, but about 360 to 460 mm (12 to 18 inches) away from your patient's eye, and look for a matching red/yellow reflex in both eyes.)

Management

Refer. It is important for the ophthalmologist to assess the cause of the problem. The patient will normally be seen within about 24 hours. Advise sedentary activities whilst waiting.

Retinal detachment

Retinal detachment is considered to be an ophthalmic urgency rather than an emergency, and the patient should be seen by the ophthalmologist within 24 hours. The notes below will help you to make a provisional diagnosis.

Predisposing causes

Ageing – the vitreous gel may undergo a benign change called syneresis, causing liquification and shrinkage of the vitreous.

Myopia – affects only 10% of the population but 40% of all cases of retinal detachment are suffered by people with myopia (Kanski and Bowling 2011).

Lattice degeneration – is a bilateral peripheral retinal degeneration that affects 8% of the adult population (Koshy 2005). Around 30% of retinal tears are lattice related and a good proportion of these are people with myopia.

Trauma – accounts for 10% of retinal detachments, and is more common in boys (Kanski and Bowling 2011).

Cataract surgery – particularly if there is a vitreous loss from a myopic eye, this may predispose to retinal detachment (Kanski and Bowling 2011).

Symptoms

- Flashing lights (photopsia) – 60% of cases of retinal detachment are preceded by flashing lights (Kanski and Bowling 2011).
- A sudden shower of red coloured or dark spots – this is a very significant symptom, usually indicating a vitreous haemorrhage caused by the tearing of a peripheral blood vessel.

- Visual field defect in one eye, often described by the patient as a 'curtain' over the vision.

Examination
- Visual acuity will be normal unless the macula area is detached.
- Check the 'red reflex'. A large detachment may be seen as a grey area.
- If the macula is off, an RAPD may develop.

Management
Don't assume that all patients with flashing lights and floaters have a retinal detachment. Ageing changes in the vitreous gel and the occasional floater may be quite harmless.

An examination of the retina, both eyes, with dilated pupils, by an ophthalmologist is recommended within about 24 hours, depending on the duration and severity of the symptoms.

In remote locations, in the event of a patient presenting with a history giving rise to a suspicion of retinal detachment and complaining of a visual field defect, who is likely to have a delayed referral, recommend immediate suspension of strenuous work activities and, when you have ascertained where the visual field defect is located (see 'Visual fields by confrontation' in Chapter 9), recommend resting on the opposite side to the visual defect to prevent or slow further detachment.

Hospital treatment may involve laser or cryotherapy to an early retinal tear or surgery to a more serious problem.

Sudden loss of vision with pain

Temporal arteritis (giant cell arteritis)
This condition is a result of a generalised inflammation of the medium and large arteries of the head and neck, which may also involve the carotid arteries and aorta. The temporal artery, which provides the blood supply to the optic nerves is commonly affected, and it follows that if the blood supply to the optic nerve is compromised, sight will be lost. This condition most commonly arises in the 60 to 75 age group, with women being more affected than men. The person may already have a documented history of hypertension, arterial disease and diabetes.

Differential diagnosis of emergency eye conditions

Symptoms

Note: This condition may initially present as an amaurosis fugax-type transient loss of vision or a sudden painless loss of vision on waking. The symptoms below may develop later.

- Headache, which may develop suddenly or come on gradually over several days or weeks. The headache may be one-sided or bilateral and get worse in the evenings.
- Tenderness of the scalp over the temporal arteries. The inflamed arteries may be visible and palpable. Brushing the hair may be painful.
- Pain in the jaw or tongue, particularly when eating or talking.
- Problems with vision, blurred vision or sudden transient loss of vision.
- The person may feel generally ill, tired, depressed, fevered, with loss of appetite and weight loss.

Examination

Check ESR, FBC, urea and electrolytes, blood pressure, urine. C-reactive protein increases in cases of inflammation and falls as the inflammation subsides. Opinion on the utility of this more expensive test is divided. Salvarini *et al.* (2002) believe this to be the most sensitive indicator of giant cell arteritis. However, Epperley *et al.* (2000) state that, although the C-reactive protein level is typically elevated in these patients, the test provides no better data than the less expensive ESR. Parikh *et al.* (2006) suggest using both tests is beneficial.

Possible complications

Complications do not usually occur if treatment is started promptly. Possible complications of untreated temporal arteritis could include:

- blindness in one or both eyes
- rarely, a cerebrovascular accident (CVA).

Diagnosis

The diagnosis is usually made by the ophthalmologist on the basis of the patient's symptoms, ESR and C-reactive protein test. Temporal artery biopsy may be undertaken but positive or negative pathological findings are not always taken as proof of the presence or absence of this condition.

Management

As this is a systemic condition, the patient should have a same-day referral to the physicians rather than to the eye department, unless the patient's vision is affected. Many of these patients also have polymyalgia rheumatica. If the patient's vision is affected, consult the ophthalmologist immediately with the results of the blood tests.

Treatment

Treatment is with oral or intravenous steroids.

Prognosis is good, as, with steroid treatment, the vision of the second eye is likely to be preserved, and the condition is self-limiting over about two years.

Optic neuritis

Optic neuritis is an inflammation of the optic nerve, usually presenting at ages 20 to 50, most commonly occurring in Caucasian women in their early 30s.

History

- Acute painless blurring of vision that may have improved over time.
- Possible history of viral illness or other neurological symptoms.

Symptoms

- Reduced vision.
- Most, but not all, patients will have pain on eye movements.
- Reduced colour vision perception in terms of 'red desaturation', in other words the colour red appears dulled in the affected eye.

Signs

- RAPD. If you are dilating patients' pupils for the ophthal-mologist to examine the retina, it is critical to check for this first and to get the ophthalmologist to double check it because of its diagnostic significance.
- A possible central loss of vision, demonstrated by a confrontation visual field test (see 'Visual fields by confrontation' in Chapter 9).
- A possibly pale optic disc on first presentation.

Management

- Steroid treatment produces a rapid improvement in the visual symptoms. The condition is strongly linked with the development of multiple sclerosis (MS) but is not a diagnostic indicator for MS, the diagnosis of which is complex.
- Ring the ophthalmologist to discuss management (but not at night).

Do remember that you will need to make sure that any patient with a sudden loss of vision or transient loss of vision is warned not to drive until investigations are complete, treatment started and they have been symptom free for a month.

Hypopyon and hyphaema

Hypopyon & hyphaema

Hypopyon

This may be defined as the presence of white cells in the anterior chamber of the eye (between the anterior surface of the iris and the posterior surface of the cornea). It may be seen as a white level within the bottom of the anterior chamber as the cells settle.

Figure 3.10

Hypopyon

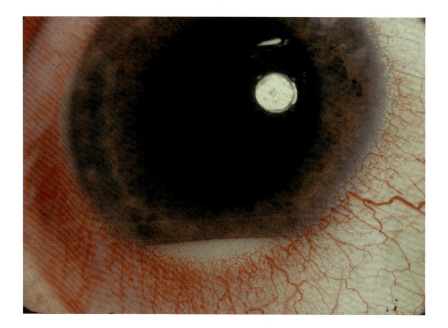

Symptoms

- Reduced visual acuity
- Usually painful

History

- There may be a previous history of, e.g. iritis or corneal ulcer.
- Patient might be a contact lens wearer.

Hypopyon is a symptom of a range of underlying conditions such as severe uveitis or corneal ulcer, all of which require emergency ophthalmic treatment.

Management

Ring the ophthalmologist (even at night).

Hyphaema

Blood visible in the anterior chamber of the eye is called a hyphaema. The hyphaema may be obvious to the naked eye or it may only be visible on slit lamp examination (microscopic hyphaema).

A blunt or penetrating injury to the front of the eye may cause

Figure 3.11

Hyphaema

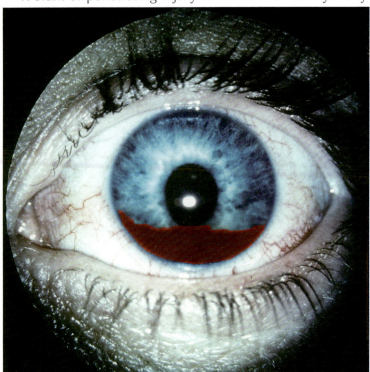

bleeding from a traumatised iris into the anterior chamber of the eye. Blood does not easily clot in the anterior chamber and further bleeding may cause the pressure in the front of the eye to rise dramatically. Untreated raised intra-ocular pressure could cause permanent visual loss.

Additionally, a large blood clot, or the presence of red blood cells in the anterior chamber may block the trabecular meshwork, causing a rise in intra-ocular pressure. A persistent blood clot in the anterior chamber may permanently stain the cornea. Most hyphaemas clear spontaneously in a few days, if the patient rests to avoid the danger of a re-bleed.

History
- Has there been any trauma?
- How was the injury caused?
- Spontaneous hyphaemas can occur with patients on warfarin but are quite rare.

Examination
- Visual acuity will be reduced.
- Check for additional injuries – a hyphaema may be present when the eye has suffered a penetrating injury. It should also be remembered that a blunt injury sufficient to cause a bleed inside the eye may also have caused retinal damage.

Management
Advise the patient against any unnecessary physical activity. If there are no other injuries, for example head injuries or penetrating eye injury, and the patient is otherwise well and in no pain, refer to the local eye department to be seen within 24 hours of the injury so that the retina can be checked for possible injury. If the patient subsequently develops any pain, they should be immediately referred to the ophthalmologist, as the intra-ocular pressure may have risen.

Treatment
Hospital treatment is likely to include:
- exclusion of any other, more serious underlying trauma
- an intra-ocular pressure check
- steroid eye drops to prevent post-traumatic iritis
- pressure-reducing eye drops, e.g. timolol maleate (Timpotol), if the pressure is raised
- advice regarding rest.

References

Bates, N. (2004). Focus on crowd control agents. *Poisons Quarterly*, Spring Supplement 5(2):6–7.

Brodovsky, S., McCarty, C. and Snibson, G. (2000). Management of alkali burns: An eleven year retrospective review. *Ophthalmology*, **107**(10): 1829–1835.

Chan, W., Michaelades, R., Ohri, H. and Towler, M. (2005). *Acute Assessment and Management of Chemical Trauma to the Eye*. Royal College of Ophthalmologists Annual Conference, Birmingham: RCO.

Dayan, M. (1996). Lesson of the week: Acute angle closure masquerading as systemic illness. *British Medical Journal*, **313**: 413–415.

Department of Health (1999). *Statement on 2 Chlorobenzyllidene Malononitrite (CS)*, London: DH.

Dua, H., King, A. and Joseph, A. (2001). A new classification of ocular surface burns. *British Journal of Ophthalmology*, **85**: 1379–1383.

Duane, T. and Jaeger, E. (1992). The retina and glaucoma. In *Clinical Ophthalmology* **3**. Philadelphia: Lippincott.

Epperley, T., Moore, K. and Harrover, J. (2000). Polymyalgia and temporal arteritis. *American Family Physician*, **62**(4): 789–796.

Fedder, I., Vlasses, P., Rocci, M., Rotmensch, H., Swanson, B., Ferguson ,R., (1984). Relationship of morphine induced miosis to plasma concentrations in normal subjects. *Journal of Pharmaceutical Science*, **73**(10): 1496–1497.

Fraser, S., Asaria, R. and Kon, C. (2001). *Eye Know How*. London: BMJ Books.

Fraser, S. and Siriwardena, D. (2002). Interventions for acute non-arteritic Central Retinal Artery Occlusion. *Cochrane Database of Systematic Reviews* 2002,1.

Fulcher, T., McNab, A. and Sullivan, T. (2002). Clinical features and management of intraorbital foreign bodies. *Ophthalmology*, **109**(3): 494–500.

Galloway, G., Wertheim, M. and Broadway, D. (2002). Acute glaucoma with abdominal pain. *Journal of the Royal Society of Medicine*, **95**(11): 555–556.

Gandhewa, R. and Kamath, G. (2005). Acute Glaucoma Presentations in the Elderly. *Emergency Medicine Journal*, **22**(4): 306–307.

Hammond, C. (2000). Disorders of the visual pathway. *Optometry*, 28 July: 28–34. Available at http://www.optometry.co.uk/clinical/details?aid = 122 (accessed 14.01.14).

Hayreh, S., Zimmerman, M., Kimura, A. and Sanon, A. (2004). Central Retinal Artery Occlusion: Retinal survival time. *Experimental Eye Research*, **78**(3): 723–736.

Kaiser, P., Friedman, N. and Pineda, R. (2004). *The Massachusetts Eye and Ear Infirmary Illustrated Manual of Ophthalmology*, 2nd edn. Philadelphia: Saunders.

Kanski, J. and Bowling, B. (2011). *Clinical Ophthalmology: A Systematic Approach*. 7th Edn. Philadelphia PA: Elsevier Limited.

Koshy, Z. (2005). Prophylaxis of Rhegmatogenous Retinal Detachment. *Focus – an occasional update from the Royal College of Ophthalmologists*, **36**, Winter.

Kotecha, A. (2002). Clinical examination of the glaucomatous patient. *Optometry*, 25 January: 34–37. Available at http://www.optometry.co.uk/ (accessed 14.01.14).

Differential diagnosis of emergency eye conditions

Krishnan, S., Roldan, C. and Das A. (2004). Retinal artery occlusion is a marker of significant carotid arteries and heart disease. *Journal of Investigative Medicine*, 52(1): 145.

Kuckelkorn, R., Schrage, N., Keller, G. and Redbrake, C. (2002). Emergency treatment of chemical and thermal eye burns. *Acta Ophthalmologica Scandinavica*, 80(1): 4–10.

Lafferty, K. (2014). Orbital Infections Treatment & Management, emedicine. Available at http://emedicine.medscape.com/article/784888-treatment (accessed 12/01/14).

MacEwan, C.J. (1999). Ocular injuries. *Journal of the Royal College of Surgeons*, 44: 317–223.

Mitry, D., Bunce, C., and Charteris, D. (2013). Anti-vascular endothelial growth factor for macular oedema secondary to branch retinal vein occlusion. The Cochrane Library. Available at http://onlinelibrary.wiley.com/doi/10.1002/14651858.CD009510.pub2/pdf (accessed 14/01/14).

National Institute for Health and Care Excellence (2012). Clinical Knowledge Summaries. Herpes Simplex – genital.

Parik, M., Miller, N.R., Lee, A.G., Savino P.J., Vacarezza, M.N., Cornblath, W., Eggenberger, E., Antonio-Santos, A., Golnik, K., Kardon, R. and Wall, M. (2006). Prevalence of a Normal C-Reactive Protein with an Elevated Erythrocyte Sedimentation Rate in Biopsy-Proven Giant Cell Arteritis. *Ophthalmology*, 113(10); 1842–1845.

Public Health England and Wales (1988). Public Health Infectious Diseases Regulation Act 1988. Statutory instrument 1546, Public Health England and Wales, London: HMSO.

Salvarini, C., Cantini, F., Boicardi, C. and Hunder, G. (2002). Polymyalgia and Giant Cell Arteritis. *New England Journal of Medicine*, 347(4): 261–271.

Skuta, G. (1994). The angle closure glaucomas. In Podos, S. and Yanoff, M. (Eds) *Textbook of Ophthalmology*. London: Mosby.

Tumosa, N. (2003). Ageing and the Eye. In Beers, M. and Berkow, M. *The Merck Manual of Geriatrics*. Available at http://www.merckmanuals.com/ (accessed 14/01/14).

Velasuoma, M., Muller, L., Gallar, J., Lambiase, A., Moilanen, J., Hack, T., Belmonte, C. and Tervo, T. (2000). Effects of Oleoresin Capsicum pepper spray on human corneal morphology and sensitivity. *Investigative Ophthalmology and Visual Science*, 41(8): 2138–2147.

UK Sepsis Trust (2014). Clinical Toolkits. Executive Summary: Emergency Department management of Sepsis. Available at http://sepsistrust.org/wp-content/files_mf/1409306430EMExecSummary2014.pdf (accessed 24.11.14).

Vernon, S. (1999). *Differential Diagnosis in Ophthalmology*. London: Manson.

Welch, L., Hunting, K. and Mawudeku, A. (2001). Injury surveillance in construction: Eye injuries. *Applied Occupational and Environmental Hygiene*, 16(7): 755–762.

Chapter 4
Major accidents and injuries

All patients within this urgent category need to be seen in the eye emergency department within 24 hours, unless otherwise stated. Management suggestions for problems occurring overnight are given below.

Accidents and injuries

Accidents and injuries

A patient may arrive in the emergency department (ED) following a severe traffic accident or major industrial injury. Obviously resuscitation and the patient's general condition take precedence. In these circumstances, where there are severe head injuries, it is not unusual for serious injuries to the bones of the orbit and ruptured globe to be present together with general skeletal and internal injuries. A senior ophthalmologist will be required as part of a multidisciplinary approach to the patient's needs.

Fractured orbital rim

Observationally, this condition is more common in men of all ages, as a result of work injuries, sport, falls, violent injuries and traffic accidents. A person with an orbital rim fracture presents following a generalised blow to the face. Crepitus may be felt around the orbital margin. Check airway, breathing and circulation and make an immediate ED referral for full examination regarding possible head injury status and possible other fractures to the skull. If there is a suspected medial wall fracture, be alert and check for rhinorrhea (indicating that a facial fracture has caused a breach in the dura mater adjacent to the nose).

If examination and X-rays reveal no other injuries, then the ophthalmic referral is within 24 hours, provided that a ruptured globe has been ruled out.

Examination

Check:

- vision
- eye movements
- RAPD (see 'Checking for relative afferent pupillary defect' in Chapter 9)
- anterior chamber
- the back of the eye by dilating the pupil.

The ophthalmologist will manage any problems with the above but is not primarily responsible for fractures of the facial bones.

'Blow out fracture' of the orbital floor

A blow out fracture of the orbital floor is usually caused when an object larger than the orbital rim hits the face, causing a sudden increase in the pressure within the orbit. Because the bones of the side wall and roof of the orbit are usually more able to withstand this pressure, the resulting fracture most often involves the floor of the orbit. Occasionally the medial wall of the orbit or rim may also be fractured. These fractures are often associated with sports injuries or fights.

Signs

- Bruising and swelling around the eye

- Oedema and occasionally subcutaneous emphysema (air in the skin which crackles when gently palpated)

- Pain on eye movement
- Enophthalmos – the eye appears smaller due to some of the orbital contents becoming displaced through the fracture site into the maxillary sinus. This symptom may develop later, as the swelling of the orbital contents following the injury subsides.

Symptoms

- There may be numbness of the lower eyelid, cheek, side of the nose and areas around the teeth in the upper jaw on the affected side.
- Sometimes a nose bleed and sensation of nasal blockage may

occur. The patient may feel tempted to blow their nose and surgical emphysema results from air being forced into the orbit from a fractured sinus. Note: If a fracture of this type is suspected, remember to advise the patient not to blow their nose as there is a possibility of not only introducing air but also infected sinus contents into the orbit.

- Double vision (diplopia) may be caused by muscle entrapment. Typically the inferior rectus muscle becomes caught in the fracture so the patient is unable to look up and down normally and double vision occurs in both these positions of gaze (see 'Checking eye movements' in Chapter 9).

Management

- Check the patient's head injury status and observe overnight if necessary.
- Carry out a CT scan of the orbital area to ascertain the extent of the injury.
- A simple fracture of the orbital floor requires referral to the ophthalmologist to check the eye for any further injury and to the maxillo-facial team.

Overnight, the ophthalmic referral can usually wait until the morning unless there is obvious eye trauma.

Women and orbital injuries

Hartzell *et al.* (1996) showed that a third of the women with orbital injuries were victims of sexual assault or domestic violence. Staff must be aware of the possibility of non-accidental eye injuries. DoH (2000) estimated that women on average experience 35 episodes of domestic violence before seeking help. DoH (2005) states that 35% of men or women being domestically abused will experience a second attack within 5 weeks, and their children may also experience direct abuse in addition to the trauma of being passive observers. All NHS Trusts should have a clearly defined and accessible domestic abuse strategy for women and men, supported by staff training.

Black eye

This is a common condition resulting from bruising following blunt trauma.

Management

The traditional treatment is application of cold compresses. Fully check the history and document an ophthalmic examination as in Chapter 2. If there is no other obvious injury or dysfunction, advise that the swelling and bruising will take at least two weeks to clear. Make an urgent ophthalmic referral so that the pupil can be dilated for a retinal check. If any other symptoms develop, such as pain or nausea, advise the patient to ring for further advice as bleeding inside the eye may lead to a sudden rise in intra-ocular pressure which should be treated as an emergency (see 'Hyphaema' in Chapter 3).

Eyelid laceration

 An ophthalmologist is required to assess and repair an eyelid laceration because of the vital function of the eyelids in providing a complete cover for the eye and evenly spreading the tear film.

 If the injury involves the nasal corner of the eye there is a possibility that the canaliculus (tear drainage tube) has been torn.

It is important to assess the severity of the injury in terms of ensuring that the cornea is adequately covered by the eyelid. If the cornea is not covered, it needs to be kept moist. Minims of normal saline can be used in the short term. If you don't have these, drip sterile saline onto the cornea with a syringe. It is likely that a patient with a severe injury will be seen by the ophthalmologist as an emergency, because of the need to exclude the possibility of a penetrating injury of the eye.

Figure 4.1

Full thickness eyelid laceration

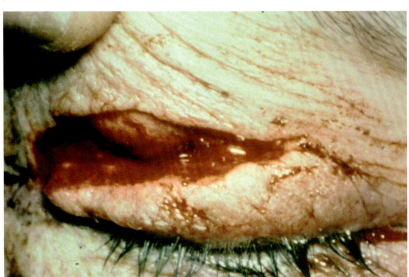

Management

- Immediate referral to ED department.
- On arrival, if the eyelid injury is severe and there is no penetrating injury to the eye, quantities of artifical tears containing carbomers (see the British National Formulary under Tear Deficiency) can be applied. Avoid greasy preparations containing white soft paraffin, which may make later examination and surgery more difficult. Try to ensure that the atmosphere around the torn eyelid and cornea remains moist by making a small 'tent' with suitable material moistened with sterile saline over the socket area.
- Prepare for a lacrimal sac washout, as, depending on the location of the injury, this may be used as a diagnostic test by the ophthalmologist to see whether the tear ducts are intact.
- During the night, if the injury to the eyelid is very severe, or an ocular penetration is suspected, ring the ophthalmologist for advice. For less severe injuries, apply a moist dressing pending evaluation by an ophthalmologist in the morning. Make sure that there is no possibility of the cornea drying out.

Subtarsal foreign body

The history is of a sudden onset of severe discomfort, particularly on blinking. Often these patients present on windy days and say 'I was just walking down the street, when suddenly…'

Symptoms

- Both eyes may be watering profusely.
- The nose may be running.
- The patient may complain of pain or discomfort when blinking.
- It will be difficult for the patient to keep the eye open.

Signs

- Visual acuity is usually normal, if the patient is able to keep their eye open long enough for you to record it.
- The eyelids may be slightly pink.

- Note: If you suspect a sub-tarsal foreign body, do not instil local anaesthetic drops to facilitate examination.

Management

- Moisten the end of a cotton wool bud with sterile saline.

- Evert the upper eyelid and remove the foreign body (see 'Everting an eyelid' in Chapter 9).
- If you can't actually see a foreign body, gently swab the upper tarsal plate with your moistened cotton wool bud.
- If the patient feels immediately better, well done! (This is why a topical anaesthetic is not instilled prior to treatment.)
- Check for corneal abrasions.
- Document what you have done and the site of the foreign body if found.
- If there is no corneal abrasion, or a superficial stain, chloramphenicol or fusidic acid 1% (Fucithalmic) may be used stat.
- If there is a large abrasion (see 'Corneal abrasion' in this chapter), or the eye looks infected, give chloramphenicol or fusidic acid 1% (Fucithalmic) ointment for five to seven days.

Advise the patient that the eye is likely to feel slightly sore for the rest of the day, and over-the-counter analgesia can be taken. By 24 hours later the condition should be substantially improved. Advise the patient to ring for further advice if the eye is not settling within this time frame.

Glue in eyes

Superglue is sometimes accidentally instilled into the eye instead of eye drops if a person who is elderly or has visual problems mistakes the superglue container for their eye drop bottle. The eyelids stick together almost immediately. It is not an ophthalmic emergency except in the sense that the patient cannot see out of their eye or eyes. The cornea is rarely damaged, as the superglue needs to be applied to a dry surface for bonding to occur.

However, if a large amount of superglue has been applied to the eye, and the eyelids are glued together, some superglue may harden behind the eyelids and in front of the cornea, causing a foreign body sensation and possibly an abrasion to the cornea.

Management

Immediate irrigation of the area with water is recommended. The eyelids can often be released using a greasy solution such as liquid paraffin or vegetable oil. Some eye departments recommend the use of an antibiotic ointment such as chloramphenicol, but given that this is more likely to cause an allergic reaction than liquid paraffin or vegetable oil, these are the preferred treatments. If gentle massage with the greasy solution does not release the eyelids, they can be kept covered with a moist eye pad, and normally open spontaneously within about four days. Only very rarely is surgical intervention required.

Problems occurring whilst removing small amounts of superglue with cotton buds soaked in liquid paraffin include loss of eyelashes as the glue is stripped away from the eyelids, and, very occasionally, the patient may develop a mild allergic skin rash in response to the glue. Make a daytime ophthalmic referral if you are unable to resolve the patient's condition.

Accidental gluing of the eyelids sometimes occurs when a distressed, struggling child has been having a brow laceration glued in an ED department. Normal practice should be to protect the eyelids by the placing of a gauze swab over the eye to protect it but this is easily dislodged by an active child. If a young child's eyelids are accidentally stuck by a stray drop of glue in these circumstances, it is unwise to wait for the lids to open over a period of days as the child may develop amblyopia of the covered eye. In this situation, apply liquid paraffin as above, and if this does not work, make an urgent (daytime) ophthalmic referral.

Paintball injury

The paint used for paintball games is not noted to be particularly toxic. Irrigate the eye and check the pH. Excess paint can be removed from the face with liquid paraffin.

Management

If the pH and visual acuity are normal, and there is no obvious eye damage, discharge the patient with antibiotic cover to prevent chemical conjunctivitis. The patient should be asked to telephone for advice if other symptoms develop or the eye does not feel completely normal after 24 hours.

Paintball injuries result from removal of the protective goggles, generally because they are splattered with paint, followed by an injury of the then unprotected eye. The real danger of a direct hit in the eye with a paintball is ruptured globe, (see 'Major Eye Injuries' in Chapter 3) and severe contusion (see 'Hyphaema' in Chapter 3). Loss of the eye or blindness may result, and an immediate ophthalmic referral would need to be made in these circumstances.

Conjunctival laceration

History

Find out exactly how the injury occurred, as you need to consider the possibility of a penetrating injury and the possibility of an intra-ocular foreign body.

Symptoms

- Mild pain
- Foreign body sensation

Examination

- Normal vision

- Red eye – possible subconjunctival haemorrhage. Be aware that a subconjunctival haemorrhage may conceal a penetrating injury.
- Laceration may be visible to the naked eye.
- Fluorescein will stain the damaged area.

Management

The conjunctiva is loosely adherent to the sclera and will heal spontaneously without suturing. Check that tetanus immunisation is up-to-date and, if the injury is minor, prescribe antibiotic ointment for five to seven days. Advise the patient to ring if any new symptoms develop, or the condition is not settling after 24 hours.

If you are uncertain that, for example, a subconjunctival haemorrhage may be concealing a penetration, or you have any other concerns, apply antibiotic ointment and advise the patient to rest at home overnight. Arrange an ophthalmic review in the morning.

Corneal abrasion

Corneal abrasion is one of the commonest acute ophthalmic presentations. There is normally a clear history of injury to the eye, which is often caused by a child's fingernail or a twig brushing the cornea.

Symptoms

- Immediate intense pain
- Watering eye
- Foreign body sensation

Major accidents and emergencies

Signs
- Red eye
- Swollen eyelids
- Blepharospasm – the patient has difficulty keeping the eye open
- Visual acuity may be slightly reduced if the abrasion is central.

Examination
- Use oxybuprocaine 0.4% eye drops or proxymetacaine 0.5% for children stat to facilitate visual acuity testing and eye examination.
- Stain the eye with fluorescein 1% eye drops to identify the abrasion.
- Do a Seidel's test to check for any potential perforation of the eye (see 'Seidel test to detect a wound leak' in Chapter 9).

Management
Minor injuries may be treated by the primary practitioner. A single application of antibiotic ointment for comfort and lubrication may be all that is needed for a minor abrasion.

Inform the patient that they will feel significantly better within 24 hours and completely better within 48 hours. The patient must seek further advice if additional symptoms develop or the condition does not improve significantly within this time period.

For large or deep corneal abrasions, Fraser (2010), after reviewing the literature, concludes that Voltarol eye drops reduce the pain caused by corneal abrasions and therefore may be instilled for pain relief. Advise regarding oral analgesia. Cycloplegics continue to be used by many practitioners for the relief of pain in corneal abrasion as they relax ciliary muscle spasm which may otherwise cause aching eye pain and light sensitivity. Carley and Carley (2001) found no good published evidence to support this practice, as the one relevant, reasonable quality study on this subject that they identify is, by their own admission, flawed. Given the difficulty of adequately controlling corneal pain and the support given by many experienced practitioners for its continued use, cycloplegia (pupil dilation) is a reasonable practice. This view is supported by Marsden (2006), who recommends cyclopentolate 1% (Mydrilate) for this purpose.

Corneal abrasions are not padded routinely. Fraser (2010) examined the literature and found that eye patching did not improve healing rates or reduce the pain of corneal abrasions.

Caution is advised with padding the young and the elderly, given the potential problems of reducing binocular vision. Marsden (2006) suggests that patients with significant pain be padded for comfort only, with the instruction that the pad can be removed if it makes the pain worse.

Mukherji *et al.* (2003) found no evidence to support the provision of tetanus prophylaxis in the ED department following superficial corneal abrasions if there was no evidence of perforation, infection or devitalised tissue. This advice is endorsed by NICE (2012).

Potential infection

Be very careful with injuries that are caused by fingernails or vegetation. A five- to seven-day course of antibiotic eye drops or ointment is indicated for all but the most minor corneal injuries.

Any abrasions with areas of loose epithelium will need expert debridement.

Overnight, treat pain as above. Apply antibiotic ointment stat. The patient should ring the local eye department in the morning for an appointment.

Corneal or conjunctival foreign body

There is usually a history of something going into the eye.

Symptoms
- Watering eye
- Foreign body sensation

Signs
- Red eye
- Visible corneal foreign body
- Normal vision (usually), but a central foreign body of
  long standing with infiltrates and oedema may affect the vision.

Typically these patients may present during the late evening or early part of the night. The reason for this is that they are less aware of the injury and discomfort whilst keeping their eyes open to concentrate on work. As they doze in a chair in the evening, or on going to bed, they may find it difficult to sleep, since the rapid eye movement (REM) stage of the sleep process will cause the foreign body to abraid the underside of the eyelid, continuously disturbing their sleep.

Figure 4.2

Corneal foreign body

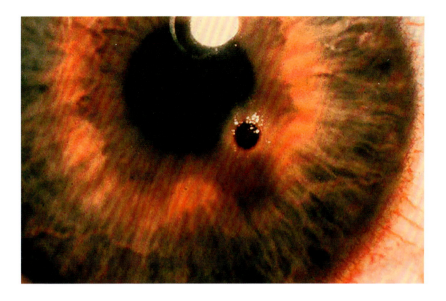

Examination

The history is very important. Did the foreign body hit the eye at
high speed, for example when hammering or chipping concrete
or using power tools? These patients may need to have their pupil
dilated for ophthalmic examination and may require an X-ray.
Was the patient wearing eye protection?

Examine the patient with a torch and exclude obvious
penetrating injury.

Management

Once a foreign body is located, you may try to flush it out of the
eye using normal saline. If this is unsuccessful, instil a local
anaesthetic drop and use a moistened cotton wool bud on the
cornea to remove superficial foreign bodies. Remember, however,
the delicacy of the cornea. The cotton bud or arrowhead swab will
cause a certain amount of corneal abrasion.

Embedded metallic foreign bodies on the cornea need expert
removal, as there is potential for permanent corneal scarring
when there is damage to the corneal stroma, which may be particularly significant in the central area of the cornea, as these white
scars may affect eyesight in the long term. Removal of the foreign

body may be relatively easy using an injection needle but rust ring
removal normally requires a slit lamp, battery-operated
disposable burr and considerable expertise. Inadequate removal
of rust will cause additional pain and delay healing. (See Chapter
7 for advice on pain management.)

Overnight, if it is not practical to remove the foreign body, there is no harm in using a very generous squeeze of antibiotic ointment, particularly under the top eyelid, to lubricate the eye and assist sleep, and applying an eyepad for comfort. Advise regarding over-the-counter analgesia. The patient can attend or ring the local eye department in the morning for an appointment for foreign body removal.

Photokeratitis ('welding flash' or 'arc eye')

Photokeratitis occurs in welders or persons who have been working close to a welding process. However, similar symptoms, as a result of other forms of ultra violet light, occur in people engaging in a variety of other activities. Personal observations of photokeratitis include: a secretary photocopying reference books all day with the photocopier lid up; sunbed misuse; exposure to snow; and sun rays reflected off the sea causing a problem for a paddler in Bournemouth Bay!

If a welder leaves off his protective goggles or shield, even for seconds, his eye is exposed to arc welding ultra violet light, which will be absorbed by the cornea and conjunctiva. Later in the day, the damaged cells will slough off, leaving nerve endings temporarily exposed, which will result in the development of acute pain. Typically this develops 6 to 12 hours after the exposure (the time varying with the degree of exposure). Generally the individual is relaxing at home or has even gone to bed before the acute symptoms develop.

Symptoms
- Intense pain in both eyes
- Photophobia
- Excessive tear secretion
- The eyelid muscles go into spasm, making it almost impossible to open the eyelids.

Signs
- Patient may look almost 'sunburned' around the face, especially the eyelids.

Examination
- Instil local anaesthetic drops, e.g. oxybuprocaine 0.4% or

tetracaine 1%, prior to examination, to relieve extreme pain and eyelid spasm.

- Instil fluorescein eye drops and use your pen torch or slit lamp with cobalt blue filter to check for punctate staining of the cornea and conjunctiva.

Management

Explain to the patient that the local anaesthetic eye drops will wear off within 10 to 20 minutes and the pain will return. Make it clear why local anaesthetic eye drops cannot be given to patients for home use. They are only used for examination purposes as in regular usage they are toxic, drying to the cornea and will impede healing (Webber *et al.* 1999). Patel and Fraunfelder (2013) found that local anaesthetic eye drops cause direct toxicity to the corneal epithelium which in turn leads to an inflammatory response in the form of infiltrate and corneal oedema. They stress the importance of adequate proper alternative analgesia to avoid topical anaesthetic abuse.

For the pain:

- Diclofenac (Voltarol) eye drops (minims) stat (or one drop four times a day for two days) will help with the corneal pain.
- No eyepads, unless requested for comfort.
- Antibiotic ointment twice a day for five days provides comforting corneal lubrication and prevents secondary infection.
- Consider pupil dilation with cyclopentolate 1% (Mydrilate) for pain management.
- Prescribe or advise about over-the-counter analgesia – possibly Ibuprofen 400 mg eight hourly, with Paracetamol between doses.

Advise the patient to contact you again if the condition is not substantially improving after 24 hours, at which stage you should consider ophthalmic referral.

Self-care

A cold compress may be soothing. Recommend two clean pillow cases, wetted under the tap, wrung out, and chilled alternately in the refrigerator (stored in a plastic bag) with a 'one on, one off rotation'. Arc eye is acutely painful in the first few hours and this helps the patient feel that they are 'actively coping'.

Educate the patient about the prevention of future problems.

Eye Emergencies: The practitioner's guide

Infections

Herpes zoster ophthalmicus (HZO, facial shingles)

Causes

HZO arises in people who have had chicken pox earlier in their lives. The latent virus becomes re-activated in the ophthalmic division of the trigeminal nerve due to normal ageing, poor nutritional status or compromised immune status. It is slightly less infectious than an attack of chicken pox, but someone with this condition should avoid mixing with immune-compromised people, babies and young children who haven't been immunised as virus particles can be transmitted from weeping lesions (Shaikh and Christopher 2002).

History

Possible flu-like illness with mild fever up to a week before the rash appears.

Figure 4.3

Herpes zoster ophthalmicus

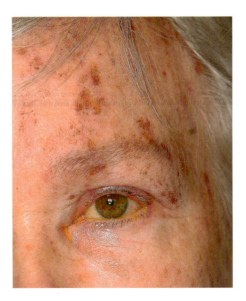

Symptoms

One-sided tingling, burning or stabbing pain around the eye followed 24 to 48 hours later by:
- red skin rash, later small clear blisters
- slight fever
- non-specific feeling of illness and tiredness
- possible blurred vision of affected eye, eye pain and red eye.

Signs

The critical sign is when the rash follows the line of the fifth cranial nerve. It appears on one side of the forehead and, if treated promptly, may involve the upper eyelid only. Typically the patient is over 60 years old.

Other signs include:

- conjunctivitis, episcleritis
- superficial punctate keratitis
- uveitis
- Shaikh and Christopher (2002) suggest that corneal involvement is present in up to 65% of patients.

After about a week, patients may develop corneal epithelial defects that look like little stars or branched lesions.

Management

The patient should be commenced on oral aciclovir (Zovirax) as soon as the rash is noted to control the progression of the disease. Alper and Lewis (2000), in a review of published research, state that prompt treatment with aciclovir with the possible addition of amitriptyline or a tricyclic drug prevents the onset of post-herpetic neuralgia.

Your patient will need a self-certificate or sickness certificate.

Patients with Hutchinson's sign – where the rash extends to the side and tip of the nose – are twice as likely to have ocular involvement, but one-third of patients without the sign are also likely to have ocular involvement (Shaikh and Christopher 2002). However, if primary physician diagnosis and treatment is prompt, very little rash may develop.

Patients with any eye symptoms at all associated with HZO should be referred to the eye department as there is a large range of potential eye complications. Overnight, advise the patient to ring or attend the eye department in the morning.

In the eye department, check:

- vision
- eye movements
- general eye health
- cornea for staining
- anterior chamber
- intra-ocular pressure.

If the nurse has any concerns at all, the patient will be referred to the ophthalmologist.

Note: Severe HZO may present in an immune-compromised patient. Full blown AIDS should be an additional diagnostic consideration.

The NHS is now offering the vaccine Zostavax to older people in the year following their 70th birthday. The vaccine will reduce the chances of people who have had chicken pox developing herpes zoster and if an attack does occur in spite of the vaccine, it will reduce the possibility of post-herpetic neuralgia.

The Department of Health research shows that Herpes zoster is more common in those aged 70 or over and the vaccination becomes less effective over the age of 80 years (DoH 2013).

Acute dacryocystitis

Dacryocystitis is generally a unilateral infection of the lacrimal sac, caused by obstruction or inflammation. It may present as an acute infection, but is sometimes chronic. It occurs at any age, but most frequently occurs in babies, due to incomplete development of the lacrimal drainage system, and older patients, who have a tendency to blockages in the lacrimal system. In the older person this may be caused by stenosis, or concretions (consisting of sulphur granules) which may block drainage.

Figure 4.4

Acute dacryocystitis

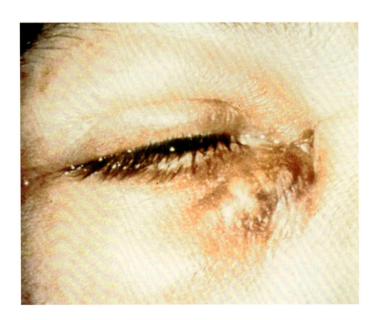

Symptoms
- Red, swollen area on the affected side, next to the nose. The swollen area may be 'pointing', looking rather similar to a boil.
- Localised pain
- Possible fever

Signs
- Eye looks watery.
- Pus may be regurgitating through the lower punctum.
- Swelling is tender to the touch.
- There may be an associated conjunctivitis.

Management
- If the patient is otherwise well, and has a normal temperature, broad spectrum oral antibiotics are indicated.
- Systemic antibiotics may be used if the condition is particularly acute, to avoid progression to a preseptal orbital cellulitis.
- Prescribe antibiotic eye drops.
- Advise regarding analgesia.
- Instruct the patient to keep the eyelids and corner of the eye clean.
- Shaw *et al.* (2010) recommend warm compresses which can also help to relieve the pain.
- A poorly child at night will need a paediatric referral. Once the infection is controlled, treatment may include teaching the parents of an affected baby how to massage the lacrimal sac to express the contents.

Differential diagnosis
A dacryocele is a collection of mucus in the lacrimal sac of a newborn baby. It is described by Kanski and Bowling (2011) as presenting in the perinatal period as a bluish cystic swelling at or below the medial canthal area. The baby has a watery eye. The cyst is filled with mucus, but may become secondarily infected. This will require an urgent ophthalmic OPD clinic referral.

Hospital treatment
- An urgent bacteriology swab should be taken from discharge present in the lower fornix.

- A 'pointing' lesion may rupture and drain spontaneously, but surgical incision and packing may be required under general anaesthetic.
- IV antibiotics may be commenced.
- Pain should be managed.
- When the condition is settled, the patient may require dacryocystorhinostomy.

Recurrent erosion of the cornea

Recurrent erosion of the cornea

A recurrent corneal erosion sometimes follows an injury, such as a corneal abrasion caused by a fingernail, bush or tree branches.

Verna (2005) describes corneal abrasions as beginning to heal from the edges, as corneal epithelial cells become flattened and move across the damaged area until it is completely covered. Healing of the abrasion is not complete until the newly regenerated epithelium is firmly anchored to the underlying connective tissue. Transient attachments are formed within one week of the injury. Normal adhesion of the healed area takes about six weeks.

Fewer tears are produced whilst sleeping and the previously abraded area is at danger of being pulled off during the healing period as the unfortunate person awakes.

History
- Previous corneal abrasion in the affected eye
- Recurrent episodes of eye pain, particularly on waking or after rubbing the eye

Symptoms
- Foreign body sensation
- Photophobia
- Blepharospasm
- Watering eye

Signs

Redness around the cornea (circumcorneal injection)

Examination
Staining with fluorescein will reveal a localised, visible disruption of the cornea which stains superficially.

Management

Emergency treatment consists of reassurance, explanation, a squeeze of antibiotic ointment into the affected eye and a primary physician or nurse practitioner referral for long-term treatment.

Viscotears during the day and Lacrilube or Simple Eye ointment at bedtime will help to reduce corneal swelling, lubricate the corneal surface and promote deeper healing of the cornea. If it fails to settle an ophthalmic referral may be necessary. Sometimes the ophthalmologist may insert a bandage contact lens. Bandage contact lenses have been demonstrated to provide a safe and effective treatment with a relatively low incidence of recurrence (Fraunfelder and Cabezas 2011).

Corneal inflammations

Corneal inflammations

Keratitis may be defined as an inflammation of the corneal epithelium, sub-epithelium, stroma or endothelium. It may be caused by an infection, or be non-infective, and has a wide range of causes, being associated with injury, contact lens wear, corneal disease, Laser Assisted In Situ Keratomileusis (LASIK) and the use of topical steroids. The sections which follow represent some of the range of infections and inflammations of the cornea that may be encountered.

Contact lens problems

Contact lens problems are likely to be caused by overuse and infection.

Overuse

All contact lens wearers should be advised to 'rest' their eyes by wearing spectacles for some period of the waking day.

However high the quality of the contact lenses, they will still inhibit oxygen supply to the cornea. Overwear will eventually result in the over-development of blood vessels at the corneal margin in an attempt to provide additional oxygen to the cornea.

The person who has been overusing their lenses will present complaining of red, uncomfortable eyes, and, following examination, needs to be advised to wear their spectacles and to consult with their optician.

Figure 4.5

Corneal neovascularisation – contact lens overuse

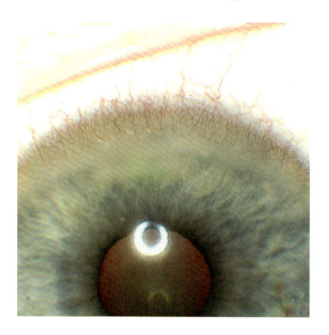

Infection

The risk of infection is increased with the use of soft contact lenses, which provide an excellent growing medium for bacteria if the lenses are not worn and cleaned according to manufacturer's recommendations. Lee and Lim (2003) maintain that silicone hydrogel lenses with their increased oxygen permeability and reduction in the risk of pseudomonas aeruginosa binding to the corneal epithelium have reduced many of the problems. However, their case report indicates that lifestyles can influence the development of problems, particularly with infection.

Fluoroquinolones have reduced hospital stays and increased the possibility of maintaining a reasonable visual outcome following severe infection, but resistant strains of pseudomonas aeruginosa are emerging.

Continued good patient education on the part of the dispensing optician is essential, with strong emphasis to the patient on urgent reporting of symptoms (see 'Bacterial corneal ulcer' in this chapter).

Giant papillary conjunctivitis

Kaiser *et al.* (2004) state that more than 95% of these patients wear soft contact lenses, have an artificial eye or have an exposed eye suture.

Symptoms
- Slightly blurred vision after inserting contact lenses
- Thick, stringy mucus discharge

Signs

- 'Cobblestone'-like lumps under the eyelids
- Conjunctival vessels beginning to encroach on the edge of the cornea

Management
Advise reduced contact lens wearing and refer the patient back to the optometrist, as factors such as edge design, surface properties, fitting characteristics, and replacement cycle can all contribute to this condition (Donshik 2003).

'Lost contact lens'
This is a common out-of-hours emergency, particularly amongst new contact lens wearers, tired people and sometimes inebriated users. The patient attempts to remove a contact lens, dislodges it from its primary position and then can't find it. The only answer is to search for the lens. Reassure the patient that, as the conjunctiva folds back on itself like a pocket, there is only so far the lens can go. Instil a local anaesthetic drop before you start looking. The eye is likely to be quite sore already from the patient's attempts to locate the lens.

- Minims of normal saline and cotton wool buds are helpful. Put plenty of the saline drops in the eye.
- Have a good look around. The most likely place for such a lens is under the top eyelid. Ask the patient to look down, evert the eyelid and pass a moistened cotton wool bud under the everted top eyelid.. Do not accidentally brush the cornea or you will cause an abrasion.
- If you put fluorescein in the eye, remember that it will stain the lens permanently, possibly making it easier to locate but the patient will need to discard the lens, if found. Mention this first.
- If you can find nothing, reassure the patient and check for abrasions that the patient may have caused to themselves and treat them accordingly. Sometimes the lens remains undetected. Ask the patient to call their optometrist or the eye emergency department in the morning if symptoms persist.

Corneal infections

Bacterial corneal ulcer

Causes

- Contact lens wearers are in the highest risk category. Failure to disinfect their lenses and lens containers, overwearing of lenses, or, in the case of disposable lenses, failure to dispose of them within the given time period, can all lead to development of bacterial corneal ulcers. Poor hand hygiene is another significant causative factor.
- Dry eyes are common in the older population and chronic blepharitis and rheumatoid arthritis are linked with dry eye symptoms. This group of patients are more prone to corneal problems.
- Eyelid closure problems, e.g. older people with bottom eyelids that droop open (ectropion), persons with Bell's palsy who are unable to blink efficiently or close their eyelids adequately and persons with eyelid scarring which interferes with normal function.
- Injury, e.g. corneal foreign body or abrasion, particularly from vegetable matter, e.g. the branch of a bush.
- 'Anaesthetic cornea', which may result from herpes zoster ophthalmicus, may cause minor injuries to go unnoticed and become infected.
- Inappropriate prescription of steroid eye drops in an effort to ease a painful red eye may cause a small infected ulcer to enlarge dramatically. Steroid eye drops are generally only used under the close supervision of an ophthalmologist.
- Patients with diabetes mellitus, dementia, chronic alcoholism and depression (Field 2005) are at greater risk of developing bacterial corneal ulcers when personal hygiene and nutrition are neglected.

Symptoms

- Severe pain
- Photophobia
- Sticky eyelids or discharge

- Ciliary flush (tiny pink/purple blood vessels visible round the cornea)

Figure 4.6

Left:
Bacterial corneal ulcer
Right:
Slit lamp view of
bacterial corneal ulcer

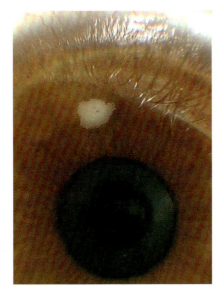
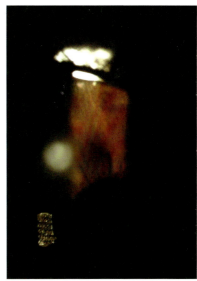

Signs

- Eyelids may be slightly red and swollen
- Vision may be slightly reduced in comparison with the other eye
- A white area may be seen on the cornea

Examination

- Use your pen torch, ophthalmoscope or slit lamp to check for the presence of a grey/white spot on the cornea.
- Instil fluorescein eye drops and, using cobalt blue filter on either your pen torch or slit lamp, check for corneal staining.
- More rarely, a hypopyon – white blood cells may be seen lying at the bottom of the anterior chamber of the eye.

Management

- Make a same-day referral to the eye emergency department. As this is a sight and eye-threatening condition, the patient who presents in the night with a hypopyon should be discussed with the ophthalmologist on the telephone.
- If there is no hypopyon, instil antibiotic ointment stat, advise regarding analgesia and make a referral to the eye emergency department in the morning.
- Following ophthalmic review, the usual treatment is with a fluoroquinolone eye drop such as ofloxacin, levofloxacin or moxifloxacin.

Marginal corneal ulcer

This is defined as a low grade response by the cornea to bacterial exotoxins released by bacteria, frequently staphylococci, colonising the eyelid margins (put simply, the patient has pre-existing blepharitis).

Symptoms
- Sore, uncomfortable, watery eye
- Foreign body sensation

Signs
- White area on corneal periphery, with slight conjunctival redness in this area
- Concurrent blepharitis and possible history of dry eyes

Examination
- Vision is normal, and the eye is only slightly red.
- A white-looking ulcer may be seen at the edge of the cornea.

Management
- Prescribe chloramphenicol ointment to eyelids. Recommend that the patient begins eyelid cleaning (see 'Blepharitis' in Chapter 5).
- Should be seen by an ophthalmologist within 24 hours of initial diagnosis for expert opinion, possible steroid eye drops or more active treatment.

Herpes simplex keratitis

Causes

The herpes simplex virus is very common. Around 80% of the population have it, possibly infected when they were children, probably from infected adults kissing them. The virus stays dormant within the body but is re-activated at times of stress or illness, often as the result of a cold, when it may reappear as a 'cold sore' near the lips. Occasionally it reappears as a very distinctive corneal ulcer.

Signs
- Red eye

Symptoms
- Photophobia

- Watering eye
- Pain or foreign body sensation
- Vision may be unaffected
- Possible previous history of herpes simplex ulcer in the same eye or cold sores

- On staining with fluorescein, a typical, branched, dendritic corneal ulcer will be revealed.

Figure 4.7

Herpes simplex keratitis (dendritic ulcer)

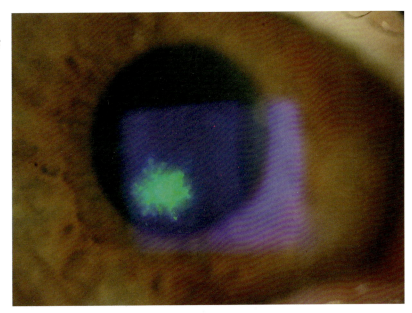

Management

The patient needs an urgent ophthalmic referral, prescription for aciclovir (Zovirax) eye ointment and a check for possible iritis, occurring secondary to the ulcer. This patient should never be prescribed steroid drops, or the ulcer will worsen and become 'geographic', spreading at an alarming rate across the cornea.

Overnight, reassurance, over-the-counter analgesia and antibiotic eye ointment stat will be adequate. Refer to the ophthalmologist within 24 hours of provisional diagnosis.

Acanthamoeba keratitis

Acanthamoeba is a protozoan that lives in infected water and soil. Corneal infection with acanthamoeba is an increasingly recognised complication of contact lens wear; if not treated promptly it may lead to corneal ulceration, and eventually to blindness (Health Protection Agency 2014) and is particularly related to poor contact lens hygiene. The acanthamoeba species can be isolated from contact lens fluid so if acanthamoeba is suspected then advise patient to retain their contact lens container and bring it to their ophthalmic consultation.

Symptoms

- Photophobia
- Pain, very acute

Signs

- Red eye
- A white area on the cornea, possibly surrounded by what looks like a white ring

Diagnosis

This is made by an ophthalmologist, following culture of corneal scrapings and cultures from contact lens cases and solutions.

Figure 4.8

Acanthamoeba keratitis

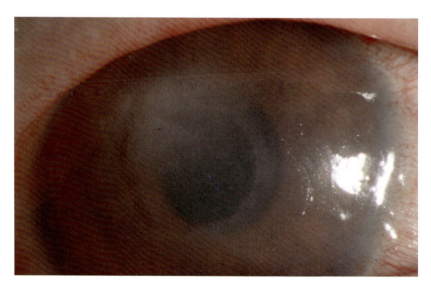

Management

Prolonged ophthalmic specialist treatment is necessary, generally with propamadine isetionate (Brolene), which eventually kills the acanthamoeba.

Overnight, if you suspect this condition, give antibiotic ointment stat, and ask the patient to ring the eye emergency department in the morning.

Uveal tract disorders

Uveal tract disorders

The 'uveal tract' is a collective term used to refer to the iris, ciliary body and choroid (hence the use of the terms anterior uveitis, posterior uveitis, iritis, iridocyclitis, cyclitis, choroiditis).

Anterior uveitis (Iritis)

Anterior uveitis is inflammation of the iris or ciliary body.

A number of systemic diseases, linked with the HLA-B27 gene are associated with the causes of uveitis. DiLorenzo (2001) stated that 19 to 88% of patients with uveitis have the HLA-B27 characteristics, depending on the population studied. HLA-B27 appears in 80 to 90% of patients with ankylosing spondylitis. Lyons and Rosenbaum (1997), in a study of inflammatory bowel disease and spondyloarthropathies noted that uveitis with spondyloarthropathies was generally anterior, unilateral, sudden in onset, and limited in duration, in contrast with patients with inflammatory bowel disease who frequently had uveitis that was bilateral, posterior, insidious in onset, and/or chronic in duration. Episcleritis, scleritis and glaucoma were also more common among patients with inflammatory bowel disease. Haroon *et al.* (2014) found that approximately 40% of patients presenting with idiopathic acute anterior uveitis have undiagnosed spondyloarthropathy. They have developed an easy to use algorithm which indicates whether referral to a rheumatologist is indicated.

In addition to the above, check for any history of respiratory symptoms (possible tuberculosis or sarcoidosis), skin problems and infectious diseases such as syphilis, shingles and cytomegalovirus, particularly in people with AIDS.

Symptoms

- Usually only one eye is affected at a time
 - Photophobia – the patient may present wearing sunglasses. Exposure to light will produce more pain
 - Aching pain, intense, located immediately behind the eye, which may feel bruised
- Watery eye, particularly on exposure to light

If the attack is severe:
 - Possible decreased vision.

Note that chronic episodes of uveitis may demonstrate fewer or none of the above signs.

Critical signs

- Small, 'muddy' looking pupil in comparison to the other eye
- Poor reaction to light
- Ciliary flush (tiny pink/purple blood vessels visible round the cornea)

Slit lamp examination

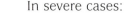
- Cells in the anterior chamber
- Blood vessels on the iris may be dilated
- A 'flare' may be seen in the anterior chamber of the eye

In severe cases:

- Keratic precipitates (KPs) – white cells may be seen sticking to the inside layer of the cornea.

- Hypopyon (white cells precipitating in the anterior chamber). This may be visible with the naked eye.

Management

The patient needs to be seen by an ophthalmologist within 24 hours. If a hypopyon is present, telephone the ophthalmologist immediately (even during the night) for advice.
Treatment will include:

- Intra-ocular pressure check
- Intensive dilation of the pupil, particularly using phenyl-epherine, to try to break down any adhesions between the posterior surface of the iris and the anterior face of the lens. Intensive pupil dilation is thought by some practitioners to be boosted by heat treatment (Ward *et al.* 2006) (see 'Application of heat to the eyelids' in Chapter 9).
- Examination of the posterior third of the eye to exclude involvement of the choroid.
- Intensive steroid drops in the acute stage, decreasing as the condition settles.
- Follow-up and intra-ocular pressure check. Occasionally the patient may require eye drops to reduce intra-ocular pressure. This is rare, but the rise may be due to the inflammatory cells produced by the iritis temporarily impeding aqueous drainage. Raised intra-ocular pressure is also associated with the strength,

frequency and duration of the steroid eye drop treatment, particularly in those with diabetes mellitus, high myopia, connective tissue disorders or a family history of glaucoma (Kaiser *et al*. 2004).

In severe cases, it may be necessary to use a subconjunctival injection of Mydricaine if the pupil remains stuck down and doesn't dilate satisfactorily. This may occasionally be combined with a steroid.

Mydricaine injections come in two strengths.

- Mydricaine One, which may be used for children, contains Atropine 0.5 mg, Adrenaline 1:1,000 0.06 ml, and Procaine 3 mg in 0.3 ml.
- Mydricaine Two contains Atropine 1 mg, Adrenaline 1:1,000 0.06 ml and Procaine 6 mg in 0.3 ml (Rahman and Pavesio 2009).

Posterior uveitis

This is an inflammation of the posterior segment of the eye. It results in inflammatory cells in the vitreous gel and has a wide variety of causes.

Associated conditions

Infections:

- viruses – cytomegalovirus (CMV), herpes simplex, herpes zoster, rubella
- bacteria – tuberculosis, brucellosis, syphilis, Lyme disease
- fungi – candida, histoplasma, cryptococcus, aspergillus
- parasites – toxoplasma, toxocara, onchocerca.

Autoimmune disorders, including:

- sympathetic ophthalmia
- systemic lupus erythematosus
- retinal vasculitis.

Malignancies, for example:

- malignant melanoma
- leukaemia.

Other conditions, for example sarcoidosis.

Symptoms

- Blurred vision – gradual onset
- New 'floaters' may be perceived in the field of vision
- Occasionally redness, pain and photophobia.

Management

The patient needs to be seen by an ophthalmologist within 24 hours.

Treatment is directed towards finding and treating the cause of the condition.

The ophthalmologist will check for: white blood cells in the vitreous, vitreous opacities, disc swelling, retinal haemorrhages or exudates.

As eye drops are only suitable for managing conditions of the anterior parts of the eye, treatment will be systemic and is likely to involve the use of steroids.

Visual perception disorders

(See also 'Sudden painless loss of vision' and 'Sudden loss of vision with pain' in Chapter 3.)

Double vision

This may be defined as seeing separate or overlapping images, instead of one single image.

Monocular double vision

Comer et al. (2007) found that, of patients presenting with double vision (diplopia) in an ophthalmic casualty department, 11.5% had monocular double vision. Surprisingly, double vision can be caused by a problem with just one eye. Ask the patient to cover one eye at a time, and check whether the double vision affects one eye. Common causes and management of this are as follows.

- An uncorrected astigmatism (abnormal contour of the cornea). Refer these patients to the optometrist to have their spectacles updated.
- Some people who are developing cataracts also complain of this, possibly even describing polyopia – a perception of multiple images. Again, an optometrist will be able to check and refer as necessary.
- Monocular double vision can also occur after cataract surgery due to malposition of the lens. You may be able to see this problem by looking into the affected eye with a good torch. Refer this person back to the ophthalmologist.

Visual perception disorders

Binocular double vision

This is caused by the eyes not working as a coordinated pair. This condition can have a sudden onset and is very distressing for the patient. The possible causes are:

- Problems with control of the eye muscles, via cranial nerves iii, iv and vi
- Head injury, cerebral tumour, benign intercranial hypertension, cerebral aneurysm, demyelination
- Problems with the eye muscles themselves, in terms of entrapment within an orbital fracture, pressure from an orbital tumour
- Micro-vascular disease – diabetes, hypertension or temporal arteritis
- Endocrine dysfunction – thyroid eye disease.

Take a full history, noting whether the condition is painful or not and whether there is any associated facial numbness. Check blood pressure and blood sugar. Note any proptosis and whether pupil reactions are equal. Check eyelid positions for ptosis or eyelid retraction. Ask about any previous episodes of diplopia. Check and document your examination of eye movements (see 'Checking eye movements' in Chapter 9).

Management

All patients with binocular diplopia require an ophthalmic referral. If an adult presents overnight, or at the weekend, in view of the 'work up' required for diagnosis, advise them to cover one eye to eliminate the condition temporarily and ask them to ring or attend the eye department in the morning for an appointment. Reassure the patient and advise them not to drive until they have been fully assessed.

Many of these people are treated with prisms in their glasses to relieve their double vision. Children's eyes are never covered, even temporarily to relieve double vision, without orthoptic management.

Within the eye department, management of diplopia will include checking the general health and symptoms as above and discussing appropriate blood tests with the ophthalmologist. Arrange an orthoptic review to see whether the double vision falls into a recognisable pattern. A quick check of the eye movement disorder may help by providing the orthoptist with useful information to help determine the patient's urgency.

CT scan and neurological referral may be necessary. Always check for third nerve palsy.

Third nerve (oculomotor) palsy

As far as eye movements are concerned, a problem with this nerve may present a confusing picture, and, depending on the severity of the problem, the patient may be unable to move the affected eye up, down or inwards. Initially they may not notice that they have double vision because of the drooping top eyelid resulting from concurrent paralysis of the levator palpaebrae superioris. You should be alerted to the potential problems by the drooping eyelid. Some patients may have a partially dilated or even widely dilated, unreacting pupil and blurred vision due to paralysis of the spincter pupillae and the ciliary muscle.

Incomplete lesions of the third cranial nerve are common within this complex condition. The patient should be referred to the ophthalmologist in the first instance, and then to the orthoptic department for accurate measurements and charting of the problem prior to consultant ophthalmologist referral.

Causes

Kanski and Bowling (2011) states the following causes of isolated third nerve palsy:

- Idiopathic – about 25% of these lesions have no known cause.
- Vascular – systemic disease such as hypertension and diabetes are the most common causes of 'pupil sparing' third nerve palsy.
- Aneurysm of the posterior communicating artery, which causes a painful palsy with pupil involvement (with or without an overt subarachnoid haemorrhage).
- Trauma – causing raised intracranial pressure.
- Miscellaneous causes such as tumours, syphilis and vasculitis.

 Be alert for a movement disorder in which the eye could be described as 'down and out', a dilated pupil on the affected side and a pain that is said to feel as if one has been hit across the back of the head with a metal shovel (thunderclap headache). Refer immediately to ED, as this could be due to a potentially life-threatening cerebral aneurysm in the occipital region (Goodwin 2006).

Migraine

It is not uncommon for patients to present complaining of an eye problem when in fact they have a migraine symptom.

Symptoms

- Classical migraine patterns may begin with a small blind area in the field of vision.
- A dazzling pattern of zig zag flashing lights may then develop, lasting 20 to 30 minutes. It is perceived as being bilateral.
- A headache might follow, but not always.

If the patient telephones, question them closely about previous possible migraine history. Even without a migraine history, if you think this is the problem, advise the person to rest quietly for an hour with their eyes closed, and give advice for self-medication should a headache develop. Advise the patient to book a primary physician appointment and ring back for further advice if the visual disorder continues.

Post-operative related eye problems

Post-operative problems

History and examination

Obtain a full history of the patient's condition and surgery. Check visual acuity and examine the eye.

Remember that any patient who has had intra-ocular surgery such as cataract extraction, retinal or glaucoma surgery may develop an acute post-surgical rise in intra-ocular pressure. The symptoms are very similar to those of acute glaucoma in terms of pain, nausea and reduced vision, and should be treated with the same urgency. (See 'Acute glaucoma' in Chapter 3.)

Other potentially serious post-operative conditions are:

endophthalmitis – an infection inside the eye itself. This is the most feared complication of eye surgery, which is thought to occur in 0.14% of cataract extractions (Kamalarajah *et al.* 2004). An acute endophthalmitis will present with pain and rapidly decreasing vision. Refer urgently for expert diagnosis.

uveitis – this is an anterior or posterior inflammation of any area of the uveal tract, which includes the iris, ciliary body and choroid which commonly occurs following intra-ocular surgery. Refer urgently for expert diagnosis.

Eye Emergencies: The practitioner's guide

Occasionally it is difficult to differentiate between the two and ophthalmic B-Scan ultrasonography might be required to provide additional diagnostic data.

Management

Always refer immediately, day or night:

- any patient who has severe post-surgical eye pain and nausea unrelieved by two paracetamol tablets or similar.

Urgent referral for:

- acute deterioration of vision.

This should ensure that you always attend to the problems listed above. Refer to the ophthalmologist or ophthalmic nurse practitioner as required.

References

Alper, B. and Lewis, P. (2000). Does treatment of acute herpes zoster ophthalmicus prevent or shorten post-herpetic neuralgia? *Journal of Family Practice*, 49: 255–264.

Carley, F. and Carley, S. (2001). Mydriatics in corneal abrasion. *Emergency Medicine*, 18: 273.

Comer, R.M., Dawson, E., Plant G., Achooon, J.P. and Lee, J.P. (2007). Causes and outcomes for patients presenting with diplopia to an eye casualty department. *Eye* 21, 413–418.

DiLorenzo, A.I. (2001). HLA-B27 Syndromes. *emedicine*. Available at http://emedicine.medscape.com (accessed 17.1.14).

Department of Health (2000). *Domestic Violence: A Resource for Healthcare Professionals*. London: HMSO.

Department of Health (2005) *Responding to Domestic Abuse: A Handbook for Healthcare Professionals*. London: HMSO.

Department of Health (2013). www.gov.uk/government/collections/shingles-vaccination-programme

Donshik, P.C. (2003). Contact Lens Chemistry and Giant Papillary Conjunctivitis. *Eye & Contact Lens: Science and Clinical Practice*, 29(1): S37-S39.

Field, D. (2005). Corneal ulcers: The social and nutritional link. *Eyelines* London: RCN. Available at http://www.rcn.org.uk/ (accessed 10.02.15).

Fraser, S. (2010). Corneal Abrasion. *Clinical Ophthalmology*. 4: 387–390.

Fraunfelder, F.W. and Cabezas, M. (2011). Treatment of Recurrent Corneal Erosion by Extended-wear Bandage Contact Lens. *Cornea*. 30(2): 164–166.

Major accidents and emergencies

Goodwin, J. (2006). Oculomotor Nerve Palsy. *emedicine*. Available at http://emedicine.medscape.com (accessed 17.1.14).

Haroon, M., O'Rourke, M., Ramasamy, P., Murphy, C. and Fitzgerald, O. (2014). A novel evidence-based detection of undiagnosed spondyloarthritis in patients presenting with acute anterior uveitis: the DUET (Dublin Uveitis Evaluation Tool). *Annals of the Rheumatic Diseases, The Eular Journal*, doi: 10.1136/annrheumdis-2014-205358.

Hartzell, K., Botek, A., and Goldberg, S. (1996). Orbital fracture in women due to sexual assault and domestic violence. *Ophthalmology*, 103(6): 953–957.

Health Protection Agency (2014). Investigation of Intraocular Fluids and Corneal Scrapings. B52, Issue 5.2, Standards Unit, Microbiology Services, Public Health England. Available at: www.hpa.org.uk/SMI (accessed 24.11.14).

Kaiser, P., Friedman, N. and Pineda, R. (2004). *The Massachusetts Eye and Ear Infirmary Illustrated Manual of Ophthalmology,* 2nd edn. Philadelphia: Saunders.

Kamalarajah, S., Silvestri, G., Sharma, N., Khan, A., Foot, B., Ling. R., Cran, G. and Best, R. (2004). Surveillance of endophthalmitis following cataract surgery. *Eye*, 18(6): 580–587.

Kanski, J. and Bowling, B. (2011). *Clinical Ophthalmology: A Systematic Approach*. 7th edn. Philadelphia PA: Elsevier Limited.

Lee, K. and Lim, L. (2003). Pseudomonas keratitis associated with continuous wear silicone-hydrogel soft contact lens: a case report. *Eye and Contact Lens: Science and Clinical Practice*, 29(4): 255–257.

Lyons, J.L. and Rosenbaum, J.T. (1997). Uveitis associated with inflammatory bowel disease compared with uveitis associated with spondyloarthropathy. *Archives of Ophthalmology*, 115(1): 61–64.

Marsden, J. (2006). The care of patients presenting with acute problems. In Marsden, J. (ed) *Ophthalmic Care*. Chichester: Whurr Publishers Ltd.

Mukherji, P., Sivakumar, A. and Mackay Jones, K. (2003). Tetanus prophylaxis in superficial corneal abrasions. *Emergency Medicine Journal*, 20: 62–64.

National Electronic Library for Health (2006). Available at www.prodigy.nhs/uk. (Accessed 30.3.06).

Patel, M. and Fraunfelder, F. (2013). Toxicity of topical ophthalmic anaesthetics. *Expert Opinion on Drug Metabolism & Toxicology*, 9(8): 983–988.

Rahman, W. and Pavesio, C. (2009). A simple technique to administer mydricaine in needle-phobic patients. *British Journal of Ophthalmology*, 93: 418.

Shaikh, S. and Christopher, N. (2002). Evaluation and management of herpes zoster ophthalmicus. *American Family Physician*, 66(9): 1723–1726.

Shaw, M., Lee, A. and Stollery, R. (2010). *Ophthalmic Nursing*. 4th edn. Chichester: Blackwell Publishing.

Titcomb, L. (1999). Mydriatic-cycloplegic drugs and corticosteroids. *The Pharmaceutical Journal,* 263(7074): 900–905.

Verna, M. (2005). Corneal Abrasion. *emedicine*. Available at http://emedicine.medscape.com (accessed 17.1.14).

Ward, B., Raynel, S. and Catt, G. (2006). The uveal tract. In Marsden, J. *Ophthalmic Care*. Chichester: Wiley.

Chapter 5
Non-urgent eye conditions

People who have had eyelid problems, for example ectropion or entropion, slightly sore eyes, or gradually fading vision over a long period of time, are clearly not emergencies, and should be treated if appropriate by primary care services or referred to the ophthalmic OPD clinic. A quick way to get to the nub of the problem when treating patients with chronic or longstanding eye complaints in an emergency department is to enquire why they came today, at this time. Some patients give seemingly endless preambles about things they think relate to a new, acute symptom. For example, a person with uncomfortable dry eyes for 18 months, may now have developed a sudden loss of vision in the right eye and assume the problems are related.

Face and eyelids

Bell's palsy

Seventh cranial nerve palsy is a post-infectious immune facial neuropathy that occurs spontaneously and is responsible for three-quarters of all facial palsies. It affects both sexes equally, and is most common between the ages of 15 and 60. Bell's palsy presents as an obvious unilateral facial paralysis (but in rare cases can be bilateral), as there are paired facial nerves, each supplying one side of the face. The symptoms are caused by inflammation of the facial nerve as it passes through the bony facial canal, which results in compression of the nerve. The cranial nerves are responsible for eye blinking and closure and facial expressions. They also control the flow of tears and saliva, the taste sensation and the function of the stapes in the inner ear.

Bell's palsy progresses from initial symptoms to maximum

facial weakness in 3–7 days. Untreated, 85% of patients begin to recover in about three weeks.

Holland and Weiner 2004 observed that the highest incidence of Bell's palsy was in the 15 to 45 age group, particularly in pregnant women. They further suggested that it was likely that the herpes simplex virus, dormant in most individuals, might be implicated in this inflammation of the seventh nerve. This has since been confirmed. Numthavaj *et al.* (2011) report that positive serology for the virus has been detected in 20–79% of patients. The onset of the facial palsy may be gradual or sudden. Tiemstra and Khatkhate (2007) stated that Lyme disease may be responsible for 25% of cases of Bell's palsy in endemic areas of North America following tick bite.

Signs

Possible facial distortion due to:

- lowering of the eyebrow due to loss of muscle tone in the affected area of the face
- difficulty closing the affected eye
- failure of the blink reflex
- ectropion (bottom eyelid hanging down)
- twitching of the affected muscles
- problems with speech clarity.

Figure 5.1

Bell's palsy
(The lower lid has lost muscle tone, and the patient is unable to close her eye completely.)

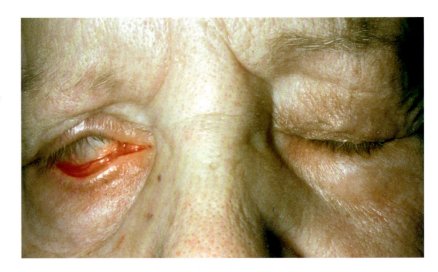

Symptoms

- Numb face and paralysis
- Dry eye

- Tears running down the face due to ectropion
- Pain and discomfort and partial paralysis around the jaw, dry mouth and alteration in taste sensation which result in difficulty eating and drinking
- Hypersensitivity to sounds and ear pain.

Examination
- Check visual acuity
- Check that a full history is obtained, as differential diagnosis can include: Lyme disease, sarcoidosis, tumour, trauma and ear infection.

Emergency management
- Give immediate advice regarding keeping the cornea lubricated, possibly using one of the carbomer group of artificial tears hourly, and a liquid paraffin ointment such as Lacrilube for use at night.
- Advise regarding taping the affected eye shut at night or use of moist eye chamber to retain the moisture in the eye. These are particularly useful if the patient has reduced vision in the other eye and may need to get up at night. Advise also regarding oral hygiene.
- Refer for ophthalmic opinion in the eye emergency department which should be carried out within one to two days regarding the possible differential diagnoses above, diagnostic tests and treatment. Aciclovir and prednisolone are being increasingly used as it is thought that the condition may be due to under-lying herpes simplex infection (Holland and Weiner 2004). Recent relevant studies demonstrate that the current practice of treating Bell's palsy with antiviral treatment plus corticosteroid leads to a slightly higher recovery rate than treating with corticosteroid alone (Numthavaj *et al.* 2011).

Paracetamol or Ibuprofen may be used for pain and reduction of inflammation.

Although the signs and symptoms of this condition are unpleasant, people of working age generally manage their symptoms well following a supportive and practical interview with a health professional, and carry on working normally.

Xanthelasma

Xanthelasma is a benign, pale, fatty lesion, occurring in the skin of the eyelids. These lesions are more common in women, peak during the 30–40s, but do tend to occur with advancing age. There are no symptoms.

As with arcus senilis, Urbano (2001) notes the strong association between xanthelasma and hyperlipidaemia, so this patient should also be screened for hyperlipidaemia.

Cosmetically, the lesion can be removed, but if the patient has hyperlipidaemia, the lesion may reduce over a period of time as a result of low fat diet and cholesterol-lowering drugs. Any referral should be via ophthalmic OPD clinic.

Demodex

This is now thought to be the cause of many presentations of blepharitis and meibomianitis. It is estimated (Sengbusch and Hausworth 1986) that about one-third of children and young adults carry the mites, but two-thirds of older people are affected, possibly because they produce more sebum, which the mites feed on. Yam *et al.* 2014 comment that demodex infestation has been found in children with refractory blepharitis, and has also been reported in adults with recurrent chalazion. They found that in a sample of 48 patients with recurrent chalazia, demodex mites were found in 35 of those examined (72.9%). Their success rate in preventing recurrence by the use of tea tree oil was 96.8%. Schachter (2014) recommends Cliradex eyelid wipes. However these, or any other tea tree eyelid wipes, are currently not available in the UK. Caution is advised as essential oils can be extremely toxic to the eye if applied incorrectly.

Blepharitis and meibomian gland disease

These are common, usually bilateral, chronic inflammatory disorders of the eyelid margins. They are usually associated with symptoms such as dry eyes, marginal ulcers, styes and chalazia (plural of chalazion, an infected meibomian cyst of the eyelid). The main causes for these conditions are:

● chronic staphylococcus infection, involving the anterior edge of the eyelid, characterised by scaling and crusting along bases of the eyelashes – often caused by a staphylococcal infection which causes inflammation of the eyelids and produces toxins which irritate the eyes. Vascular changes at the eyelid margin may be noted.

- seborrheic blepharitis – associated with dandruff of the scalp producing greasy, flaky scales at the base of the eyelashes, causing blockage of meibomian gland orifices.
- Infestation of the eyelash follicles with demodex mites.

Meibomianitis is caused by blocked meibomian glands which may cause meibomian cyst formation. This results in an unstable tear film, causing what McCulley and Shine (2003) term 'evaporative dry eye'. Meibomian gland dysfunction (MGD) is considered to be the leading cause of dry eye disease throughout the world (Nichols *et al.* 2011).

Symptoms
- Chronically irritating gritty eyes, particularly in the evenings
- Eyelid margins may be crusted in the mornings
- Visual acuity may be mildly affected as a result of the deficient tear film accompanying dry eyes

Figure 5.2

Blepharitis
(note the dilated, plugged orifices of the meibomian glands)

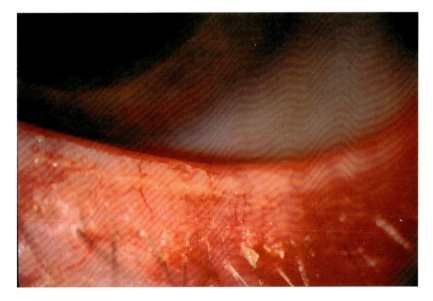

Signs
- Crusting can usually be seen on the eyelash margins
- Eyelids are red
- Conjunctiva may look red
- On slit lamp examination, meibomian gland ducts on the eyelid

margin may be enlarged and 'weeping' or even blocked with plugs of mucus.

- Frothing of the tear film seen on the eyelid margins.

Management

- Check for marginal ulcers, or associated acne rosacea and refer to an ophthalmologist to be seen in the eye emergency department in one to two days if appropriate.
- Remember patients with deep-seated staphylococcal infections may require systemic antibiotics for at least six weeks to control the infection.
- Advise regarding reducing or discontinuing the use of eye make-up, which clogs the orifices of the meibomian glands.
- Stress good personal hygiene and the importance of treating dandruff of the scalp.
- Lid hygiene twice a day is essential. Historically this consisted of cleaning the base of the eyelashes thoroughly with a sodium bicarbonate solution or baby shampoo diluted 50:50 with water, applied with a cotton wool bud. It is washed away using further cotton buds dipped in cool boiled water. For people with busy lifestyles, proprietary 'lid scrubs' or solutions are available at optometrists and pharmacies, though these tend to be expensive. Some patients use eye make up removal pads successfully to keep their lid margins clean and comfortable. Stress the importance of continuing the cleaning regime to control the condition.
- Advise applying warm compresses to the eyelids, using pads of cotton wool and very warm water twice a day. Gentle massage following the warm compresses will help break down mucus plugs in the meibomian glands. An eye bag or mask filled with linseed is now available and microwaved for 1 minute to warm it up. This is expensive but less labour intensive. A recent trial by Bilkhu et al. (2014) has demonstrated the efficacy of the eye bag, particularly if used on a regular, long-term basis. Research by Olson et al. (2003) has demonstrated an increase in tear film lipid layer thickness following treatment with warm compresses in patients with meibomian gland dysfunction. Nichols et al. (2011) recommend increasing dietary intake of omega-3 fatty acids and, in more severe cases, topical azithromycin. However this is expensive and best left to the ophthalmic department.

Artificial tears specific to MGD are now available; these aim to replace the lipid layer.

- Chloramphenicol ointment or fusidic acid 1% (Fucithalmic) may be massaged into the eyelids twice a day, using a clean finger, for ten days (after lid hygiene) if necessary. Generally this condition should be dealt with at primary care level. In persistent cases the chloramphenicol ointment or fusidic acid 1% can be used every night for one month.

Molluscum contagiosum

This is a highly infectious viral skin condition characterised by clusters of small pink, pearly-looking spots. It usually affects school-aged children, sexually active young adults, and immuno-compromised individuals. It is benign and self limiting and most cases spontaneously resolve within 6 to 9 months (Lee & Schwartz 2010). It is caused by pox virus, and is spread by direct skin or mucous membrane contact and indirect contact, such as sharing baths and towels.

Management

When molluscum contagiosum lesions occur around the eyelids they can cause a toxic conjunctivitis. If a person with molluscum contagiosum lesions around the eyes develops follicular conjunctivitis, make a routine referral to the ophthalmic OPD clinic for evaluation, as incision and curettage or cryotherapy may be required. However there is not enough evidence to show that any particular treatment is effective for treating molluscum infection (Van der Wouden et al. 2011).

Lid lumps

Our faces are exposed to the sun throughout our lives and basal cell carcinomas (BCCs) and squamous cell carcinomas occur quite frequently around the eyelids as a result of this. BCCs are relatively common, with the incidence varying depending on the region of the world, with the highest rate of 1 to 2% per year noted in Australia. It is estimated by Zak-Prelich et al. (2004) that BCC incidence is increasing by 5% annually due to social and environmental changes. A more recent article by Arits et al. (2011) has demonstrated a 7% increase for both genders over the last two decades.

You may discover little painless eyelid growths whilst examining the eyelids for something entirely different. If unsure of the diagnosis, these patients should be referred to the ophthalmic OPD clinic.

Lice

Infestations of lice are sometimes present in the eyelashes and eyebrows

Symptoms

Red, very itchy eyelids.

Signs

Eggs in various stages of development, sticking to the eyelashes

Management

Direct removal of most of the lice from the eyelids using fine forceps, under slit lamp microscopy, is normally undertaken in the eye emergency department. This may be followed by the application of petroleum jelly to the base of the eyelashes twice a day for a week, which is effective in eradicating the lice but does not destroy the eggs (Ma and Vano-Galvan 2010). The patient is then reviewed, as further removal of lice and applications of petroleum jelly may be required.

Advise that following specific treatment of the infected areas of the body, bedlinen and clothes should be washed and dried on a hot cycle.

A person presenting with lice in the eyelashes may also have a pubic, and possibly a hair, infestation. Provide advice for dealing with these. It is accepted practice to refer the patient to the Sexually Transmitted Diseases clinic for a check for the possibility of other infections and expert advice regarding treatment for possible contacts. For the eyelashes, refer to the local eye emergency department via telephone, during the daytime.

Ticks on the eyelids

Ticks may carry Lyme disease and febrile illnesses, which are passed into their hosts if the tick is left in place for longer than about 24 hours, or an inept removal is attempted, causing them to vomit their stomach contents into their host. Referral to the local eye emergency department is the safest way to handle this problem, as the staff are likely to have specialist tick removal forceps.

History and examination

Document a full eye examination and history. Record how long the tick was in situ.

Management

You should never:

- crush, squeeze or puncture the tick
- apply substances to smother it
- burn it
- twist or jerk the tick to get it out
- use bare hands to handle it.

Within the eye department the specialist tick-removing forceps should be used following the manufacturer's instructions. If these are not available, or cannot be used due to the position of the tick, use Mathalone forceps. Grasp the tick firmly across its head and mouth to prevent it regurgitating its stomach contents into its host as close to the patient's skin as possible. Pull out the tick without squeezing the tick's body or twisting – there may be some resistance. If mouth parts are left in the wound, removal, where possible, is advisable.

Provide chloramphenicol ointment for use three times a day to the wound site for three to five days. If the tick is fully removed discharge the patient. If some mouth parts remain in the wound, follow up in three to seven days.

All patients should be advised to seek a medical opinion promptly if they develop any rash around the original bite, joint pains, flu-like symptoms or facial palsy within 3 to 30 days. They must explain that they have had a recent tick bite. Clinical studies have shown that more than 96% of patients who find and remove an attached tick will not contract Lyme disease (Stanek *et al.* 2012).

Stye (external hordeolum)

This is an acute staphylococcal infection in the sebaceous glands of Zeiss and Moll at the base of the eyelashes or in the hair follicle itself. It may be associated with blepharitis.

Symptoms

Eyelid lump, redness, swelling or tenderness of several days' duration.

Eye Emergencies: The practitioner's guide

Figure 5.3

Stye

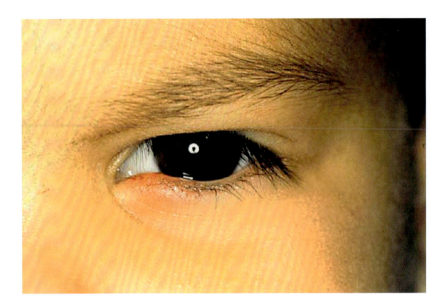

Signs

Visible or palpable lump within the eyelid, often pointing around an eyelash follicle. In early cases, a lump may not be identified. The eyelid is slightly swollen and acutely tender.

Examination

A stye is located on the lid margin.

Management

- Warm compresses, twice a day and more frequently if possible.
- Systemic antibiotics are rarely used unless the patient is developing cellulitis. Antibiotic ointment is sometimes prescribed to smear on the affected eyelid to prevent the infection spreading to other eyelash follicles. The condition will resolve spontaneously in one to two weeks without treatment.
- Removal of an eyelash associated with the stye is rarely carried out as it is exquisitely painful and the replacement lash may grow at an odd angle, causing further problems.
- Check for possible diabetes in people who have recurrent infections and refer back to their primary physician for further management.

Chalazion (internal hordeolum)

A chalazion is a lump in the eyelid that forms owing to the blockage of a meibomian gland. In the chronic stage meibomian gland secretions become retained due to the blockage of the duct, causing a localised swelling, which may need incision and curettage.

Figure 5.4

Chalazion
(eyelid everted)

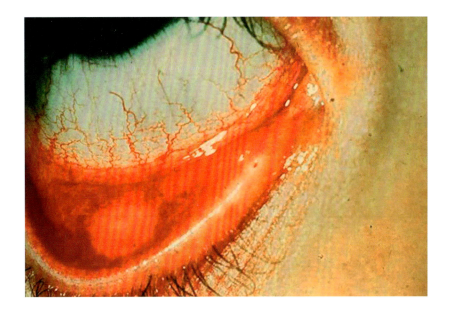

Signs

In the acute stage there is localised redness and swelling of the lid due to acute infection. On examination there is a swelling of the eyelid arising from behind the lid margin. Eversion of the eyelid may show a yellow area deep in the tarsal plate.

Symptoms

These range from a mild sensation of discomfort to pain, together with distorted vision if a very large cyst is pressing on the cornea.

Management

Be aware that eyelid malignancies are occasionally confused with meibomian cysts.

In the acute stage, recommend warm compresses to soften the secretions that are blocking the duct. Antibiotic ointment may be prescribed.

After the inflammation has subsided, the patient with a chalazion may be left with a lump. The patient can be advised to contact the surgery in 8 to 12 weeks if the lump remains, with a view to referral for incision and curettage. Given time, the lump will subside, but patients may not be willing to wait longer than a few months.

Eye Emergencies: The practitioner's guide

Note: If the eyelids are very swollen the patient could be developing preseptal cellulitis and may need treatment with systemic antibiotics.

Trichiasis

Trichiasis is inflammation of the eyelids from chronic blepharitis often leads to eyelashes growing unevenly.

Symptoms

Sore, slightly red eye with normal vision.

Trichiasis is a problem that affects older patients. It causes no problems unless the affected eyelashes begin to brush against the eye, in particular the cornea. This causes progressive discomfort, and chronic corneal abrasions, which may become infected, leading to corneal ulceration.

Management

- Always advise people with blepharitis on routine eye care. Problems with ensuing dry eyes and trichiasis may thus be considerably reduced.
- If an eye examination discloses an unevenly growing eyelash(es), do not routinely epilate unless the front of the eye is being abraded. Check the eye with fluorescein stain first. Epilation just might cause the eyelash(es) to grow back at a worse angle.
- Initially, mild trichiasis can be managed by epilating any lashes abrading the cornea and asking the patient to come back if there are further problems. Check that it is a true trichiasis and not as a result of the eyelid turning in (entropion).
- More severe problems should be referred to the Ophthalmic OPD Clinic. Cryotherapy, argon or diode laser or electrolysis treatment may be tried.
- A small number of people have very severe problems that do not respond well to the above treatment. Ideally, they need regular weekly or fortnightly appointments with an optometrist or ophthalmic nurse to epilate the eyelashes using a slit lamp and fine forceps.
- Once the offending eyelashes have been removed, any abrasions resulting from trichiasis should be treated with a short course of antibiotic ointment.

- Check whether the patient has dry eyes, which tend to accompany this condition. Treat appropriately with artificial tears.

Conjunctival problems

Note that only acute exacerbations of the milder allergies are dealt with in this section. Persons with atopic keratoconjunctivitis or vernal keratoconjunctivitis are likely to present with more acute symptoms, mild visual disturbance, photophobia, eyelid eczema, purulent discharge, punctate staining of the upper part of the cornea and possibly papillae at the limbus. 'Out of hours' they can be treated with mast cell stabilisers and antihistamines, but need to be reviewed in the long run in the ophthalmic OPD clinic.

Acute allergic conjunctivitis

This alarming condition generally affects children or young adults who have a previous history of allergies.

History

Children often present as having been 'just playing' when the symptoms began. Careful questioning will probably elicit details of exposure to a specific allergen such as animal fur, dust or pollen.

Symptoms

- Itching and burning sensation of one or both eyes
- Normal visual acuity
- Watering eye(s)

Signs

Sudden onset of mild to severe swelling of the eyelids and the conjunctiva. The swelling of the conjunctiva is alarming and tends to look pale and jelly-like.

Management

- Reassure the patient or parents.
- Advise the parents that the child needs to be bathed or showered to remove traces of allergen, particularly from the face, hair and hands, and that they should provide clean clothes.

- These presentations are often in the evening, so a stat dose of oral chlorphenamine (Piriton), depending on the age of the child, followed by an early night, is helpful.
- Cold compresses will reduce the swelling and itching.
- Advise the patient or parents to contact their surgery in the morning if the condition is not settling, as possible longer-term treatment may be required. (See below.)
- Over-the-counter medications may be the most cost-effective initial treatment for the adult patient. Artificial tears may be suggested for comfort. The local pharmacist is able to help with advice regarding a range of non-prescription eye drops and systemic antihistamines. If this is unhelpful, further medical advice may be sought through an appointment at the surgery.
- If you decide to supply medication yourself, be particularly cautious with young children. Many topical antihistamines are unsuitable for children under 7 or even 12 years of age. There are also precautions regarding pregnancy and breastfeeding.

Perennial allergic conjunctivitis

Perennial allergic conjunctivitis, which affects adults or children, is an allergic reaction to substances present all the year round, such as animal fur, feathers, moulds and droppings of household dust mites.

History

The eyes are uncomfortable and slightly itchy throughout the year. The condition may worsen in the spring, as a result of pollens, and during autumn due to decaying vegetation and moulds. There may be a history of other concurrent allergies, for example rhinitis, eczema or asthma. Consider the possibility of an allergy to eye make-up.

Symptoms

Symptoms are bilateral.
- Normal visual acuity
- There may be slight photophobia, particularly in the early morning
- The eyelids may be swollen, and the eyes are itchy
- Watering eyes

Signs

- Slightly red eyes
- Watery or stringy discharge
- Fine papillae may be present
- No corneal involvement

Management

- Topical – mast cell stabilisers or antihistamine, or combination eye drops. (If prescribing mast cell stabilisers advise the patient that they take at least a week to work.) Olopatadine (Opatanol) is a particularly useful eye drop for children as it is a twice daily instillation and works well as a combination of antihistamine and mast cell stabiliser.
- Advise regarding the control of potential allergens within the environment.
- Advise regarding changing, reducing or discontinuing eye make-up.

'Hay fever' conjunctivitis

This condition occurs mainly in the spring and is associated with pollens. It is bilateral.

Symptoms

- Normal visual acuity
- Itchy, gritty feeling in both eyes
- Running eyes, with watery mucus discharge
- Sneezing and itchy, running nose

Signs

- Red eyelids
- Conjunctival redness
- Fine papillae
- Cornea not involved

Management

- Topical – mast cell stabilisers or antihistamine, or combination eye drops.
- Advise regarding systemic antihistamines.

Eye Emergencies: The practitioner's guide

Bacterial conjunctivitis

Symptoms
- A sticky, purulent discharge from one eye, with possible slightly later spread of symptoms to the other eye.
- Itchy, irritating superficially sore eye, sometimes there is a complaint of foreign body sensation.
- Vision normal, patient otherwise feeling well.

Signs
- The eye and insides of the eyelids are red, with the redness particularly concentrated on the conjunctiva lining the eyelids.
- Petechial haemorrhages (tiny red spots as a result of micro haemorrhages) may be seen on the tarsal plates when you evert the eyelids.

Examination
Check for corneal involvement by staining with fluorescein. (If the cornea is involved, seek ophthalmic advice, as infections such as gonorrhea cause a very acute conjunctivitis.)

Management
Treatment is normally provided in terms of antibiotic eye drops – either chloramphenicol or fusidic acid 1% (Fucithalmic). Bacterial conjunctivitis is said to be 'self-limiting'. It would go away without treatment within two weeks. In British society it is customary to treat to prevent others getting infected and to reduce the period of quarantine from school for children to 24 hours.

A recent Cochrane Review paper (Sheikh and Hurwitz 2006) states that the use of antibiotics in this condition is associated with a significant improvement in rates of clinical and microbiological remission. As the condition may become bilateral, some practitioners recommend treating both eyes with antibiotics from the outset. If the condition does not clear within a couple of weeks, a referral to the local eye emergency department for review is indicated.

Fusidic acid 1% (Fucithalmic), or no treatment, is applicable for pregnant or nursing mothers. Fusidic acid 1% is particularly useful for children, as it only needs to be applied twice a day. However it is usually only effective on staphylococcal aureus infections.

Advise the patient to bathe the eye regularly with warm water and moistened cotton wool swabs to remove any crusts from the eyelids. Clean paper tissues should be used to mop away any tears or discharge and carefully disposed of. Stress the importance of personal hygiene, such as handwashing, using own face cloth, towel and soap so as not to spread the infection to others.

Parents of children with conjunctivitis should be advised to keep them away from school or nursery until the eyes are free of discharge, as the disease is highly contagious.

Viral conjunctivitis

The patient may give a recent history of having had an extremely sore throat, cough and cold.

Symptoms
- The affected eye(s) feel very sore
- Watery discharge, resembling straw-coloured tears.
- Photophobia
- Visual acuity may be a little reduced if the central cornea is affected.

Figure 5.5

Viral conjunctivitis

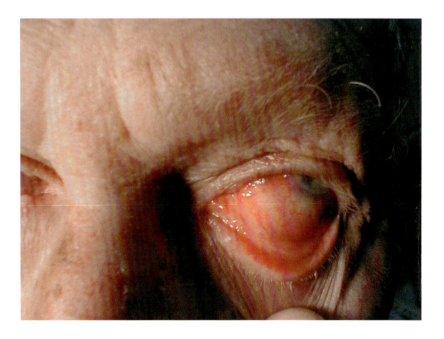

Signs
- Swollen eyelids

- Follicles
- Red eye, possibly with petechial subconjunctival haemorrhages
- Possible pseudomembrane formation under the eyelids
- Possible central corneal involvement in terms of small circles of epithelial keratitis
- Pre-auricular lymph nodes palpable (just in front of the ear)

Management

Sympathetically explain that the condition typically gets worse for the first four to seven days but will resolve without treatment in three to six weeks and that antibiotics will not help. This person is miserable with this acutely uncomfortable condition. However, the eye emergency department would generally not want to see these patients unless referred by the primary practitioner, as their attendance could cause a departmental epidemic. The patient may need a sickness certificate for up to two weeks.

Supply artificial tears for comfort. Some patients find oral analgesia helpful. Low dose topical steroids provide a little relief but should only be supplied by an ophthalmologist. Steroids are generally used only if there is corneal involvement and these have to be used cautiously because if the causative virus is herpes simplex then steroids could make it worse. There is some discussion in the literature (Shiney *et al.* 2000) regarding the use of topical ketorolac (Acular) instead of artificial tears to relieve the pain, but this is not a mainstream approach.

Chlamydial (inclusion) conjunctivitis

The patient frequently presents with a history of having been treated ineffectively for conjunctivitis over a number of weeks with at least two different antibiotics. The patient is sexually active and may disclose some genito-urinary irritation and discharge or have no symptoms at all. Chlamydia trachomatis is an intracellular parasite and has its own DNA and RNA; as a result it is more closely related to bacteria than to viruses. Serotypes D-K produce adult inclusion conjunctivitis (Marsden 2006). It is more common in the 16 to 25 age group.

Symptoms

- Uncomfortable eye
- Sticky discharge

Signs

- Occasional mild swelling of pre-auricular lymph glands
- Red eye
- Characteristic large follicles and papillae under upper and lower eyelids
- Possible corneal involvement

Management

Unlike bacterial or viral conjunctivitis, this condition is not self-limiting. If you suspect that a patient may have this condition, refer to the ophthalmologist for specialist bacterial, viral and chlamydial swabs. If there are genito-urinary symptoms, refer also to the Sexually Transmitted Disease clinic. Treatment is with systemic antibiotics usually prescribed by the genito-urinary clinic after taking swabs. It is not usual to treat the eye topically.

Differential diagnosis guide: types of conjunctivitis

SIGN/SYMPTOM	BACTERIAL	VIRAL	ALLERGIC	CHLAMYDIAL
PAIN	Foreign body sensation	Very sore & uncomfortable	Bilateral, intense irritation & itching	Foreign body sensation and irritation
DISCHARGE	Mucopurulent present on waking	Watery eyes, straw-coloured tears	Clear, watery, stringy	Mucopurulent
EYELIDS	Crusted, mild swelling	Swelling when severe	Moderate swelling, red	Crusted, mild swelling
CONJUNCTIVA	Red, particularly inside lids	Follicles, diffuse redness & possible chemosis (swelling)	Papillae, diffuse redness & possible chemosis (swelling)	Red, follicles, particularly inside lids
CORNEA	Clear	Small corneal opacities	Clear	Generally clear but may get SPK
ANTERIOR CHAMBER	Clear	Clear	Clear	Clear
IRIS	Normal	Normal	Normal	Normal
PUPIL	Normal reaction	Normal reaction	Normal reaction	Normal reaction
SYSTEMIC SYMPTOMS	Nil	Possible upper respiratory tract infection	Possible hay fever, nasal symptoms, asthma, eczema	Genito-urinary symptoms may be present. Sexually active.

Conjunctival cyst

Causes

These may be observed following eye surgery, but also occur spontaneously.

Symptoms

- Mild, superficial discomfort
- Possible watery eye

Signs

Clear, fluid-filled cyst on the eye itself, or inside the eyelids. This may be an incidental finding during an eye examination.

Treatment

Topical lubricants may be tried if this is the person's presenting symptom. Practice experience shows that the cysts generally recur if incised with a needle. In the past cysts were occasionally excised. There is little researched, best treatment advice published, but Hawkins and Hamming (2001) report a technique using cauterisation under slit lamp visualisation, which they describe as quick and effective.

Subconjunctival haemorrhage

Subconjunctival haemorrhage is bleeding under the conjunctiva, which is only loosely adherent to the eye and is a common presentation within general practice and minor injuries departments. Seewoodhary (2003) stresses the importance of carefully assessing every patient, as it is occasionally a symptom of a more serious condition. It is known that degenerative changes occur in superficial conjunctival vessels which makes them bleed more readily in response to some of the stressors indicated below under 'history'.

Symptoms

- Normal visual acuity
- Possible mild irritation
- Generally symptomless

Signs

- A flat, bright red haemorrhage under the conjunctiva

● Very occasionally the haemorrhage may be more severe and form a dark red mass under the conjunctiva which protrudes over the lower lid margin.

Figure 5.6
Subconjunctival haemorrhage

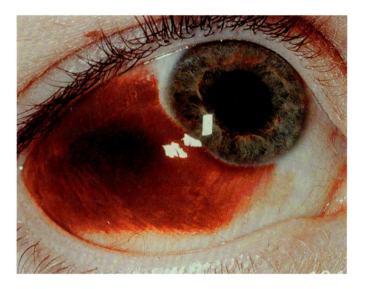

History
● Coughing, straining, vomiting
● Trauma
● Hypertension
● Bleeding disorder
● No obvious cause
● Degenerative changes in conjunctival blood vessels
● Occasionally, viral conjunctivitis, e.g. enterovirus 70
● Secondary to medicines, e.g. aspirin or warfarin

Examination
Check blood pressure unless traumatic. If it is raised, re-check after ten minutes. Examine the eye with torch or slit lamp. You should be able to see the edges of the bleed. If not, check the ocular movements to rule out retro-bulbar haemorrhage and check for any discomfort or double vision.

Management
Where no trauma is involved there is no ocular treatment. If the blood pressure is raised refer to the practice nurse for a further check. If the blood pressure is already being monitored by the general practice, send a letter for information but ask the patient

to get their blood pressure re-checked at the surgery if very high.

Where trauma is involved, unless it is very superficial according to the history and examination, the patient should see an ophthalmologist. The reason for this is that a bullous subconjunctival haemorrhage may conceal a scleral perforation. Local exploration of a wound involving the conjunctiva may be necessary. This would be carried out by an ophthalmologist at the slit lamp. It will also be necessay to dilate the pupil to examine the back of the eye to look for signs of contusion or perforation.

If the patient has suffered major trauma and there are bilateral subconjunctival haemorrhages, particularly when it is not possible to see the posterior limit of the haemorrhage, a fractured base of skull must be considered. Make head injury observations and refer swiftly to general ED department.

Recurrent subconjunctival haemorrhages could be a result of:
- fragile blood vessels if the recurrence is in the same place
- diabetes – check blood glucose.
- a clotting disorder, in which case blood screening investigations need to be arranged by the patient's general practice.

Management
Reassure the patient that the condition will resolve in about two weeks but may appear to get worse initially as the blood spreads underneath the conjunctiva and changes colour as a result of natural dispersal processes. If necessary, arrange appropriate referral for further investigations.

Concretions

Figure 5.7

Concretions

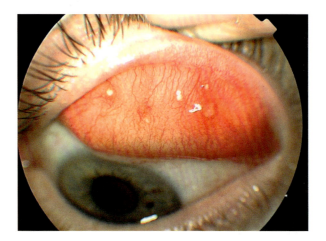

Conjunctival concretions are small white or cream inclusion cysts inside the upper or lower eyelids filled with keratin and epithelial debris. They used to be thought of as a calcium deposits. Concretions are often chance findings during examination of the conjunctiva, or are sometimes responsible for a patient's complaint of a scratchy foreign body sensation. They are more frequently noticed in the ageing eye and are possibly linked with chronic inflammation.

Symptoms
- Irritating eye
- Eye may be painful or red.

Examination
- Examination of the upper and lower tarsal plates shows either white concretions or crystal-like concretions.
- Cornea may be abraded.

Management
- Concretions are not removed unless they are poking through the conjunctiva and providing symptoms.
- If they are scratching the cornea, they may be simply removed after the application of topical anaesthetic eye drops, with an injection needle of appropriate size.

Pinguecula

A pinguecula is a harmless raised yellow growth arising from the conjunctiva. They are often present in older patients who have been exposed to sunshine. They present symmetrically, at about 3 o'clock on the nasal side of both eyes and there may be a corresponding smaller pinguecula at 9 o'clock on both eyes.

These are normally asymptomatic, unless one has become slightly more elevated, causes mild irritation and the patient suddenly notices it, and attends wanting a diagnosis.

Management

Management comprises reassurance. Most older people have pingueculae. An inflamed, uncomfortable pinguecula may require a short course of steroid drops and should be seen in the eye emergency department within a few days.

Pterygium

A pterygium is a triangular, benign vascular lesion arising from the conjunctiva. It is more common in people whose occupations have caused them to be exposed to a lot of ultra violet light, for example roofers or people from sunny climates.

A pterygium is a progressive condition, becoming thick, fibrous, and containing many blood vessels. Over a period of time, it may grow across the cornea, obscuring the pupil and interfering with the eyesight.

Symptoms

An uncomfortable eye, with a mild foreign body sensation.

Signs

A triangular lesion which may or may not have begun to encroach on the cornea.

Management

Management comprises reassurance. Artificial tears may be supplied if there is mild discomfort. Ophthalmic OPD clinic referral is not required unless the pterygium is encroaching on the cornea. It is not normally removed unless beginning to disturb the vision by its encroachment or as a result of disturbing the visual axis

Pigmented conjunctival lesions

These can be congenital, acquired, benign or malignant. They should not normally present at an ED department but may be noted as part of a careful eye examination. Pigmented lesions are common in dark-skinned populations.

Management

Bearing in mind that primary acquired melanosis is a potential malignancy, any new or changing melanotic lesion in any individual needs an evaluation. An ophthalmic OPD clinic referral needs to be made via the general practice.

Scleral problems

Episcleritis

Between the sclera and the conjunctiva lies the episclera, which sometimes becomes inflamed. The causes of episcleritis are not identified in many individuals, but in others it may be linked with gout, autoimmune disorders such as rheumatoid arthritis and bowel disorders, syphilis and tuberculosis. The condition tends to be recurrent, affecting generally only one eye at a time. It affects men and women of any age but appears to be more common in women in their 30s and 40s.

Symptoms
- Red eye
- Aching
- Slight watering
- Occasionally photophobia
- Visual acuity is normal

Examination
- There is a localised 'pink/purple' cluster of dilated blood vessels visible on the episclera.
- Sometimes there is an accompanying translucent nodular swelling.

Management

It is important to differentiate episcleritis from scleritis, which is more serious. Episcleritis is a benign condition, often not treated, as the attacks generally settle in about two weeks. Treat initially with lubricants.

Occasionally the ophthalmologist will prescribe steroid or NSAID eye drops if if is uncomfortable and not settling.

Scleritis

Scleritis is an inflammatory connective tissue disorder of the conjunctiva, sclera and episclera which is generally associated with systemic disorders such as sarcoidosis, systemic lupus, systemic vasculitis and rheumatoid arthritis.

The condition may present in the anterior or posterior section of the eye, and may affect one eye or both. If it is not treated promptly, it can cause severe damage to the eye.

Eye Emergencies: The practitioner's guide

Symptoms

Symptoms have a gradual onset which includes:

- constant, severe, boring pain, spreading to the head and face and waking the patient at night
- photophobia
- watering eye.

Signs

- Red eye(s) – often an intense red/purple/bluish appearance
- Possible slight decrease in vision
- The eye may be tender on palpation. Ask the patient to look down, and gently palpate the upper eyelid.

History

Check for underlying systemic illness.

Examination

- A slit lamp examination, if possible
- Intra-ocular pressure check

Management

Urgency will depend on the severity of the eye condition, so you will need to present a good evaluation when making your referral to the eye emergency department. The ophthalmologist may use one to two drops of phenylepherine in the affected eye to make a diagnosis. Engorged vessels caused by episcleritis will blanch, but, in scleritis, the vessels remain dilated (Patel and Lundy 2002). The ophthalmologist will also make an examination of the posterior segment of the eye via dilated pupil.

Treatment will include diagnosis and management of the systemic condition and local steroids to the eye. The ophthalmologist may make a clinic referral for more complex multidisciplinary management. This is not considered to be an emergency during the night.

Other presentations

Arcus senilis

Arcus senilis

This is a circular white/yellow lipid deposit at the edge of the cornea. It is symptomless and benign.

It is more common in older people, affecting 75% of those aged over 75 (Urbano 2001). It used to be considered to be a marker for potential raised cholesterol and coronary heart disease. However, Urbano (2001), after studying the research, concluded that arcus senilis provided no more information about mortality risk than age does. Leichter *et al.* (2013) have demonstrated a link between arcus senilis and hyperglycaemia in older patients so if you do notice this in a patient, it is good practice to suggest a cholesterol and blood sugar check anyway. There is no other treatment.

Dry eyes

This is tear insufficiency associated with ageing and a variety of systemic diseases.

Causes

Dry eyes are caused by a deficiency in any of the layers responsible for tear production.

- Post-menopausal women are more predisposed to the condition, which is also associated with inflammatory disorders and autoimmune conditions.
- It may be idiopathic – not associated with any systemic disease.
- It may be drug induced by, e.g., beta-blockers, tricyclic anti-depressants, oral contraceptives and phenothiazines.
- The patient may have Sjogren's syndrome – associated with arthritic joints and dry mouth.
- Vitamin A deficiency.

Symptoms

Symptoms of this problem may be worse than the clinical presentation.

- Scratchiness or gritty sensation, particularly on waking.
- Excessive tearing due to reflex tearing – the eyes may be particularly sensitive on hot, dry days, or in smoky atmospheres.
- Air conditioning, low humidity and exposure to the elements may worsen the complaint.

- Usually bilateral.
- Patients may complain of transient blurred vision.

Examination and diagnosis
- Make a general examination of the eye with a torch or slit lamp.
- Pay particular attention to the eyelids. People with meibomianitis are predisposed to developing dry eyes.
- Observe for mucus strands and debris in the tear film.
- Stain with fluorescein and check the tear break-up time.

It is important to identify the predisposing cause of the problem. Patients with chronic meibomianitis are likely to suffer from deficiencies in the lipid layer of the tear film.

Management
Ocular lubricants (artificial tears), for example hypromellose, should be used as necessary to symptomatically reduce the discomfort and irritation of this condition. These and more expensive preparations are available over-the-counter at the chemist.

For very dry eyes, solutions without preservatives are superior, but are more expensive. Preservatives can cause additional irritation in an already sensitive eye so preservative-free solutions should be considered if the patient needs to use lubricants more than six times a day.

Laser pointer problems
Over recent years concerns have been expressed by the general public regarding the use of laser pointers and their potential for damaging the eye. The published medical literature contains one report of what appears to have been a determined self-inflicted injury. A study by Robertson *et al.* (2000) is able to offer the reassurance, based on research findings, that 'the risk to the human eye from transient exposure to light from commercially-available laser pointers seems negligible'.

Management of such a complaint is therefore aimed at reassurance. This is not an ophthalmic emergency. However, a persistent complaint of sudden visual dysfunction would need to be investigated.

References

Arits, A., Schlangen, M., Nelemans, P.J. and Kelleners-Smeets, N.W. (2011). Trends in the incidence of basal cell carcinoma by histopathological subtype. *Journal of the European Academy of Dermatology and Venereology,* 25(5): 565–569.

Bilkhu, P.S, Naroo, S.A. and Wolffsohn, J.S. (2014). Randomised masked clinical trial of the MGDRx eyebag for the treatment of meibomian gland dysfunction-related evaporative dry eye. *British Journal of Ophthalmology*, 98: 1707–1711.

Hawkins, A.S. and Hamming, N.A. (2001). Thermal cautery as a treatment for conjunctival inclusion cyst after strabismus surgery. *Journal of American Association for Pediatric Ophthalmology and Strabismus*, 5(1): 48–49.

Holland, J. and Weiner, G. (2004). Recent developments in Bell's Palsy. *British Medical Journal*, 329: 553–557.

Lee, R. and Schwartz, R.A. (2010). Pediatric molluscum contagiosum: reflections on the last challenging poxvirus infection, part 1. *Cutaneous Medicine for the Practitioner*, 86(5): 230–236.

Leichter, S., Johnson, J., Ammerman, M. and Egbert, S. (2013). The Associations of Arcus senilis with Age and Metabolic Abnormalities. *Journal of Diabetes & Metabolism*, 4(8): 2155–2156.

Ma, D.-L. and Vano-Galvan, S. (2010). Infestation of the eyelashes with Phthirus pubis. *Canadian Medical Association Journal*, 182(4): 10.1503.

Marsden, J. (2006). *Ophthalmic Care*. Chichester: Whurr Publishers Ltd.

McCulley, J. and Shine, W. (2003). The meibomian gland, blepharitis and contact lenses. *The Eye and Contact Lenses: Science and Clinical Practice*, 29(1) (Suppl. 1): 593–595.

Nichols, K.K., Foulks, G.N., Bron, A.J., Glasgow, B.J., Dogru, M., Tsubota, K., Lemp, M.A., and Sullivan, D.A. (2011). The International Workshop on Meibomian Gland Dysfunction; executive summary. *Investigative Ophthalmology & Visual Science* 52: 1922–1929.

Numthavaj, P., Thakkinstian, A., Dejthevaporn, C. and Attia, J. (2011). Corticosteroid and antiviral therapy for Bell's palsy: A network meta-analysis. *BMC Neurology*, 11(1). Available at: www.biomedcentral.com/1471-2377/11/1

Olson, M., Korb, D. and Greiner, J. (2003). Increase in tear film lipid layer thickness following treatment with warm compresses in patients with meibomian gland dysfunction. *Eye and Contact Lens Science and Clinical Practice*, 29(2): 96–99.

Patel, S. and Lundy, C. (2002). Ocular manifestations of auto immune disease. *American Family Physician*, 66(6): 991–998.

Robertson, D., Lim, T., Salomao, D., Link, T., Rowe, R. and McLaren J. (2000). Laser pointers and the human eye. *Archives of Ophthalmology*, 118(12): 1731–1732.

Schachter, S. (2014). A different approach to treating demodex blepharitis. *Optometry Times*. January 3rd.
Available at: Available at http://optometrytimes.modernmedicine.com/ (accessed 10.02.15)

Seewoodhary, R. (2003). Subconjunctival haemorrhage: Implications for ophthalmic nursing practice. *Ophthalmic Nursing*, **7**(1): 10–14.

Sengbusch H., and Hausworth, J. (1986). Prevalence of hair follicle mites, demodex folliculorum and demodex brevis in a selected human population in Western New York, U.S.A. *Journal of Medical Entomology*, **23**(4): 384–388.

Sheikh, A. and Hurwitz, B. (2006). Antibiotics vs placebo for acute bacterial conjunctivitis. *Cochrane Database of Systemic Reviews*, 2006, **2**.

Shiney, Y., Ambati, B. and Adamis, A. (2000). A randomised double masked trial of topical Ketorolac versus artificial tears for the treatment of viral conjunctivitis. *Ophthalmology (Rochester and Hagerstown)*, **107**(8): 1512–1517.

Stanek, G., Wormser, G.P., Gray, J. and Strle, F. (2012). Lyme borreliosis. *The Lancet*, **379**(9814): 461–473.

Tiemstra, J., and Khatkhate, N. (2007). Bell's Palsy: Diagnosis and treatment. *American Family Physician*, **76**(7): 1000–1002.

Urbano, F. (2001). Ocular signs of hyperlipidaemia. *Hospital Physician*, November: 51–59. Available at http://turner-white.com (accessed 16.06.07).

Van der Wouden, J.C., Van der Sande, R., Van Suijlekom-Smit, L., Berger, M., Butler, C.C. and Koning, S. (2011). Cochrane Review: Interventions for cutaneous molluscum contagiosum. *Evidence-based Child Health: A Cochrane Review Journal*, **6**(5): 1550–1599.

Yam J., Tang B., Chan T., Cheng A., 2014. Ocular Dermodicidosos as a risk factor of adult recurrent chalazion. *European Journal of Ophthalmology*, **24**(2): 159–163.

Zak-Prelich, M., Narbutt, J. and Sysa-Jedrzejowska, A. (2004). Environmental risk factors predisposing to the development of basal cell carcinoma. *Dermatologic Surgery* **30**(2) (Suppl. 2): 248–252.

Chapter 6
Drugs commonly used for acute eye conditions

When drugs are administered into the eye they are absorbed either through the cornea or the conjunctiva, to the inner structures of the eye and then to the systemic circulation. Some of the drug will drain into the naso-lacrimal duct and be absorbed directly into the systemic circulation via the nasal mucosa (Waller *et al.* 2005). When a drug is ingested, the products of digestion are passed into the portal circulation from the gut to the liver for metabolism, reducing the amount of drug entering the systemic circulation. This is known as reduction in bioavailability. Being absorbed straight into the systemic circulation. Eye medication avoids this first pass liver metabolism. It is important to bear in mind that although the drug concentration within an eye drop may be generally low, it still has the potential to cause systemic side effects, particularly in small children. It is therefore sensible to follow the Medicines Optimisation Guidelines (NICE 2015, in press) and only prescribe or supply under protocol when absolutely necessary.

To reduce the risk of systemic side effects, Andrews (2006) suggests occluding the naso-lacrimal duct or simply closing the eye for 60 seconds after instillation of eye drops. Patients should be encouraged to report any side effects, as often they will not associate systemic complaints with eye medication.

General principles

Patients should be advised to:
- wash their hands before instilling eye medication
- only use treatment prescribed for them
- complete the course of treatment given
- throw away any unused medication
- leave at least five minutes between eye drops if instilling more than one eye drop

- use the eye drop first and eye ointment last if combining therapy
- use a clean tissue to blot away excess drops and not a used handkerchief
- keep eye drops in the fridge if required by the manufacturer.

Pregnancy and lactation

Pregnancy and lactation

Because eye preparations are absorbed systemically there is a potential risk to the unborn foetus and to breast-feeding babies. Titcomb (2004) has drawn up general principles when prescribing eye drops or ointment to pregnant or lactating patients.

- Avoid drugs whenever possible especially in self-limiting disorders.
- Only prescribe when the risk to the mother outweighs the risk to the foetus.
- Avoid eye preparations preserved with mercurial salts.
- Give the lowest effective dose for the shortest possible time.
- Reduce systemic absorption by punctual occlusion and blowing nose after application.

In breast-feeding mothers:

- the infant should feed immediately before the dose.
- if drugs are taken that are not compatible with breast feeding, the milk should be expressed and discarded.
- recommence breast feeding after a safe period, e.g. four times the drug elimination half life.

It could be argued that avoiding all drugs in pregnancy is the favoured option. However, this is not necessarily a practical option in some cases (Briggs *et al.* 2014). The prescriber or supplier of medication needs to consider the best interests of the mother and share knowledge about the particular medication required, outlining any potential risk to the foetus or newborn and so allowing an informed choice to be made.

Eye drops and contact lens wear

Contact lens wear

It is generally not good practice to continue wearing contact lenses while having topical treatment for an eye condition. Some drugs and preservatives can accumulate in soft contact lenses and cause toxic reactions (BNF 2014). This may not be such a problem

Drugs commonly used for acute eye conditions

for daily disposable contact lens wearers but should be avoided in extended wear lenses. The eye problem may well have been caused by contact lens wear in the first place and therefore part of the treatment would be avoiding contact lens wear for a period of three to four weeks or longer. It may also be worth bearing in mind that some systemic medications can affect the eye surface or tear quality.

Gas permeable lenses are not affected by topical eye drops and there may be some cases where topical treatment is extensive and contact lens wear could be resumed when the eye is more comfortable, for example in iritis when treatment continues usually for four to six weeks.

Take care when instilling fluorescein sodium dye, used for the detection of corneal abrasions or lesions, as a soft contact lens will stain bright yellow and cannot be salvaged.

Acute glaucoma

Acute glaucoma

Acetazolamide (Diamox) is one of the most significant oral or IV drugs in emergency eye care. The formation and secretion of aqueous humour by the ciliary body is a complex process in which the enzyme carbonic anhydrase plays an important role. Acetazolamide is a member of a small group of drugs known as carbonic anhydrase inhibitors. Systemically it produces a slight diuresis and it is also used in the treatment of epilepsy.

In acute glaucoma, acute secondary glaucoma or raised intra-ocular pressure in the adult, 500 mg of acetazolamide is given IV as a stat dose. This is followed by oral doses of 250 mg, but no more than 1g total should be given over 24 hours (rarely, a consultant ophthalmologist may prescribe an additional dose if complete sight loss is threatened). Diamox is not recommended for long-term use. It has many quite serious side effects, the commonest, including tingling of hands and face, nausea, confusion and sleepiness, being the least serious.

Apraclonidine 0.5% (Iopidine) eye drops act on the adrenoreceptors in the walls of the blood vessels of the eye, causing them to narrow, restricting the blood supply and thus reducing the amount of aqueous humour being secreted. Apraclonidine's effects on the intra-ocular pressure are

143

measurable within an hour, and it continues to work for three to five hours following the instillation of a single drop.

Pilocarpine hydrochloride (2 and 4%) is a miotic, a parasympathomimetic drug which produces a small pupil thus pulling the trabecular meshwork open to facilitate aqueous drainage from the anterior chamber of the eye. It is not readily absorbed into the circulation of the eye until the intra-ocular pressure begins to fall.

Antibiotics

Antibiotics

These are preparations that are prescribed to combat bacteria that are sensitive to their effects and are either bacteriostatic or bacteriocidal.

Bacteriostatic preparations inhibit the growth or reproduction of bacteria by hindering bacterial protein production, DNA production and cell metabolism, giving the body's immune system the opportunity to generate a lethal response to the bacterial attack. In higher doses, most of these drugs are also bacteriocidal. **Bacteriocidal** preparations kill bacteria.

Chloramphenicol is a bacteriostatic, broad spectrum antibiotic used widely for minor eye infections and bacterial conjunctivitis. Use eye drops either four times a day for five to seven days or two hourly for two days then four times a day for five days if the eye is very sticky. Over-the-counter chloramphenicol drops are now available as Optrex Infected Eyes. Chloramphenicol ointment is used more for chalazia, corneal abrasions or keratitis where a lubricating effect is also required. Use chloramphenicol ointment twice a day, three times a day or four times a day, depending on the condition.

Fusidic acid 1% (Fucithalmic) is a bacteriostatic preparation used mainly for children where a twice-a-day dose is preferable. It is useful mainly for bacterial conjunctivitis where the causative organism is staphylococcus aureus (Titcomb 1999, Kanski and Bowling 2011). It is supplied in a tube, and is a transparent, non-greasy viscous preparation which 'melts' on contact with the eye. Dosage is usually twice a day for five to seven days.

Fluoroquinolones (Ciprofloxacin and Ofloxacin) are bacteriocidal agents used commonly for contact lens induced corneal ulcers under ophthalmic supervision and are particularly

Drugs commonly used for acute eye conditions

effective against pseudomonas infections (Grahame-Smith & Aronson 2002). Bacterial ulcers are usually treated hourly, even overnight in some instances, with drops and ciprofloxacin is also available in ointment form for night time usage. Treatment is reduced when the ulcer shows signs of healing, usually after 48 hours.

Neomycin is bacteriostatic with some bacteriocidal effect, although Grahame-Smith and Aronson (2002) admit that the bacteriocidal effect is through a mechanism not yet fully understood. It is generally used in combination with a steroid to treat marginal ulcers or keratitis. However, it can be useful in treating young children with pseudomonas infections, as fluoroquinolones are not recommended under the age of four years.

Antihistamine and mast cell stabilisers

Name of drug	Antihistamine (AH) or mast cell stabiliser (MCS)	Frequency of dosage	Age recommendation	Cost per 10 ml
Antazoline sulphate (Otrivine Antistine)	AH	TDS	Over 12 years	£2.35
Sodium chromoglicate (Opticrom, Haycrom)	MCS	QDS	No age given	£1.84
Lodoxamide (Alomide)	MCS	QDS	Over 4 years	£5.21
Azelastine (Optilast)	AH	BD to QDS for a maximum of 6 weeks	Over 4 years but longer periods over 12 years	£8.00
Olopatadine (Opatanol)	combined	BD for a maximum of 4 months	Over 3 years	£9.36
Nedocromil sodium (Rapitil)	MCS	QDS	Over 6 years	£5.72
Emedastine (Emadine)	AH	BD	Over 3 years	£14.62
Ketotifen (Zaditen)	Combined	BD	Over 3 years	£15.78
Epinastine hydrochloride (Relestat)	AH	BD for a maximum of 8 weeks	Over 12 years	£19.80

BNF 2014. Medicines optimisation. In press.

Antihistamine eye drops such as antazoline sulphate (Otrivine Antistine) are available over-the-counter and can be very effective in relieving itching from allergies. For longer-term treatment, mast cell stabilisers are advised and should be started before the allergy season starts as they take at least a week to take effect. Mast cell stabilisers act by inhibiting the release of inflammatory mediator cells (Grahame-Smith and Aronson 2002). Alternatively, olopatadine blocks the histamine receptors to ease the symptoms of allergy and is useful because it can also be prescribed for children over the age of three (BNF 2014).

Antivirals

Antivirals

Aciclovir is the first choice treatment for herpes simplex infections. It is a guanosine derivative which has a high specificity for herpes simplex and varicella-zoster viruses but the herpes simplex virus is more susceptible to aciclovir than varicella-zoster (Rang *et al.* 2011). It is used five times a day for ten days, but if further treatment is needed then the treatment should be reduced to three times a day as aciclovir is quite toxic to the eye and can cause keratitis. For herpes zoster ophthalmicus, oral aciclovir 800 mg five times a day for seven days is the usual dosage. It can safely be used in children but if given orally the dosage should be reduced (BNF 2014).

 ## Steroids

Steroids

Steroid eye drops should only be used under the supervision of an ophthalmologist. The BNF (2014) advises three main dangers.
- A 'red eye' may be due to herpes simplex virus and steroids will make the condition much worse.
- They can lead to 'steroid-induced glaucoma'.
- They can lead to the development of cataracts.

Prolonged use of steroids can also lead to thinning of the cornea and sclera.

Prednisolone 0.5% (Predsol) is the mildest steroid eye drop and often used in episcleritis if the condition will not settle using lubricants. It is usually four times a day for a week, then twice a day for a week.

Betamethasone (Betnesol) is the next strength and is used less commonly but is often used in combination with neomycin post-ophthalmic surgery.

Dexamethasone (Maxidex) is used for mild to moderate cases of iritis (anterior uveitis) and can be used as frequently as hourly to reduce inflammation initially and then gradually tailed off over five to seven weeks.

Prednisolone 1% (Predsol Forte) is used in moderate to severe iritis and would be used as frequently as Dexamethasone (Maxidex).

Lubricants

Lubricants

A number of products are available to lubricate the eye. Generally when the eye feels and looks dry and there is an absence of tears then products such as hypromellose may be sufficient. However, when the tear quality is poor, meaning the mucin or oily layer is deficient, then a gel replacement from the carbomer group is preferable such as GelTears, Liposic, Liquivisc or Viscotears.

If the patient complains of a watery eye with a gritty sensation this is often an indication of poor tear quality rather than a lack of tear production. Whatever product is chosen, regular use is vital, sometimes as often as hourly until the corneal surface is lubricated and the eye comfortable. Twice a day is not enough! It is often a question of patient choice as patients find some lubricants more beneficial than others. Carmellose sodium (Celluvisc) is very effective as a short-term solution to corneal dryness but its cost deters long-term use. Sometimes a few weeks of carmellose sodium is enough to get the patient back on course so that they can return to their usual lubricant. There are also products available to help replace lipid content within the tear film such as Systane Balance among others.

Artificial tears without preservative may be necessary in sensitive patients. These include single dose hydroxyethylcellulose (Artificial Tears) minims, carbomer (Viscotears) single dose and carmellose sodium (Celluvisc). In addition an increasing number of topical lubricants now have excipients which neutralise on contact with the tear film, for example, Oxyal. To maintain ocular lubrication overnight, ointments such as liquid paraffin (Lacrilube or Simple Eye ointment) can be helpful.

Local anaesthetics

All topical anaesthetic eye drops take about one minute to have an effect but some last longer than others and this length of effect determines their usage.

Tetracaine 0.5 and 1% lasts about 20 minutes and is used for cataract extraction operations and subconjunctival injections

With oxybuprocaine 0.4% the anaesthetic effect lasts for about 15 minutes, and it is used for foreign body removal or procedures such as irrigation, syringing of the naso-lacrimal duct or measuring intra-ocular pressure.

Proxymetacaine hydrochloride 0.5% (proparacaine) has an anaesthetic effect of about 15 minutes and is said to sting less than other local anaesthetics so is particularly useful for children. It also comes in minims mixed with fluorescein for eye examination or measuring intra-ocular pressure.

Lignocaine hydrochloride 4% (lidocaine) has an anaesthetic effect of about 30 minutes and minims mixed with fluorescein are available for measuring intra-ocular pressure.

Lidocaine hydrochloride, proxymetacaine hydrochloride and tetracaine should be avoided in pre-term neonates because of the immaturity of their metabolising enzyme system (BNF for Children 2014)

Local anaesthetics delay corneal wound healing and can cause keratitis (Bartlett and Jaanus 2001) so should never be given to patients to take home.

Pupil dilators

Anatomy and physiology

The iris has two muscles:

- a sphincter muscle which runs in a circular mode around the pupil and is responsible for constriction
- a radial dilator muscle which dilates the pupil.

The sphincter muscle is controlled by parasympathetic fibres of the oculomotor (third cranial nerve) and the dilator muscles by sympathetic fibres from the ophthalmic branch of the trigeminal nerve (fifth cranial nerve). The pupil can be dilated by enhancing the action of the dilator muscle or blocking the action of the

Drugs commonly used for acute eye conditions

sphincter muscle.

An eye drop which produces mydriasis dilates the pupil. For some treatment or examination purposes, it is also necessary to paralyse the ciliary muscle, which controls the focusing power of the lens. This effect is called cycloplegia.

Parasympatholytics and antimuscarinic eye drops

Tropicamide, cyclopentolate, homatropine and atropine block the action of the sphincter muscle.

Tropicamide 0.5% or 1% takes only 20 to 40 minutes to dilate the pupil, has both mydriatic and cycloplegic effects and is short acting, relatively weak and wears off after six hours. It is particularly useful for fundal examination of the eye. It stings on instillation.

Cyclopentolate 0.5% or 1% (Mydrilate) takes 30 to 60 minutes to widely dilate the pupil and is a stronger and longer-lasting mydriatic and cycloplegic than most of the other preparations (6 to 24 hours). Hence its frequent use as a treatment for ocular conditions such as anterior uveitis where it is necessary to produce both pupil dilation and cycloplegia for pain relief. Patients find cyclopentolate painful on instillation.

Homatropine 1% or 2% takes 30 to 60 minutes to dilate the pupil and its mydriatic and cycloplegic effects last for one to three days. It is used as treatment for iritis, corneal abrasions or other eye conditions where the pupil must be kept dilated for longer periods of time. It is less painful on instillation, but has largely been replaced by cyclopentolate in clinical use.

Atropine 1% takes 30 to 60 minutes to dilate the pupil, produces strong cycloplegia and its effects can last for as long as five to seven days. For this reason it is therefore only used in conditions such as severe iritis where prolonged pupil dilation is needed. It is rarely used routinely, as it can produce quite severe skin rashes following instillation and has potentially serious systemic side effects.

Sympathomimetic eye drops

Sympathomimetic eye drops cause mydriasis by enhancing the action of the dilator muscles within the iris. Therefore, for maximum pupil dilation, a parasympatholytic and a sympathomimetic are often used together.

Phenylephrine 2.5% or 10% takes about 20 minutes to dilate

the pupil and can last up to ten hours, so it is only used when the pupil must be fully dilated prior to eye surgery, when parasympatholytics and antimuscarinic drugs are not having a good effect, or when particularly strong pupil dilation is required (for example to break down posterior synechiae (adhesions) between the posterior surface of the iris and the anterior surface of the lens in anterior uveitis). Phenylephrine has a vasoconstricting effect which can be useful in the diagnosis of episcleritis or scleritis. It should be used cautiously in patients who have heart disease or high blood pressure (use 2.5%), as side effects can include cardiac arrhythmias, hypertension and coronary artery spasm (BNF 2014 and Sweetman 2004).

Pupil dilation

People with dark irises are more resistant to pupillary dilation as the pigment adsorbs the drug (Waller *et al.* 2005) and persons with diabetes are often similarly difficult to dilate. Patients should be advised not to drive after dilation. Andrew (2006) advises waiting one to two hours for the eye drop effects to wear off, but this clearly depends on which eye drops have been used and how susceptible the patient is to the medication. Many will find that their near vision is impaired for several hours and that they are acutely photophobic.

General side effects of mydriatics and cycloplegics are transient stinging and raised intra-ocular pressure. Allergic reactions are rare but can occur with cyclopentolate, homatropine and atropine (BNF 2014).

Dilating eye drops can cause an attack of acute glaucoma in certain patients so should be used with caution, especially in patients with a history of glaucoma. This pertains to patients with narrow angle glaucoma where dilating the pupil may block the drainage angle and trabecular meshwork. It is good practice to check that the anterior chamber is deep before dilating the pupils.

Diagnostic eye drops

Diagnostic eye drops

Fluorescein sodium minims or fluorets can be used in primary practice to diagnose corneal or conjunctival abrasions. Within an ophthalmic department they are also used for Seidel's test and to

Drugs commonly used for acute eye conditions

measure intra-ocular pressure using Goldman applanation tonometry. Use fluorescein sparingly as it can mask the appearance of fine detail if slit lamp examination is required. If you suspect that swabs for chlamydial conjunctivitis may be needed then do not use fluorescein as it negates the test results, not only for your patient but for the whole of the test batch.

Rose Bengal is a pink dye which shows up degenerated or damaged cells on the surface of the eye. It is not commonly used now, as it is extremely uncomfortable for the patient.

References

Andrew, S. (2006). Pharmacology. In Marsden, J. (2006). *Ophthalmic Care.* Chichester: Whurr.

Bartlett, J. and Jaanus, S. (2001). *Clinical Ocular Pharmacology*, 3rd edn. Oxford: Butterworth Heinemann.

Briggs, G.G., Freeman, R.K. and Sumner Y.J. (2014). *Drugs in Pregnancy and Lactation: A Reference Guide to Fetal and Neonatal Risk.* 10th rev edn. Philadelphia PA: Lippincott Williams and Wilkins.

British National Formulary (2014). London: BMJ Publishing Group.

British National Formulary for Children (2014). London: BMJ Publishing Group.

Grahame-Smith, D. and Aronson, J. (2002). *Oxford Textbook of Clinical Pharmacology and Drug Therapy*, 3rd Edn. Oxford: Oxford University Press.

Kanski, J. and Bowling, B. (2011). *Clinical Ophthalmology: A Systematic Approach.* 7th edn. Philadelphia PA: Elsevier Limited.

National Institute for Health and Care Excellence (2014). *Medicines optimisation.* In press.
http://www.nice.org.uk/guidance/indevelopment/gid-cgwave0676/documents

Rang, H., Dale, M., Ritter, J. and Moore, P. (2011). *Pharmacology* 7th edn. Edinburgh: Churchill Livingstone.

Sweetman, S. (2004). *Martindale: The Complete Drug Reference*, 34th edn. London: Pharmaceutical Press.

Titcomb, L. (1999). Topical ocular antibiotics: Part 1. *The Pharmaceutical Journal*, 263: 298–301.

Titcomb, L. (2004). Topical ophthalmic antimicrobial agents in pregnancy and lactation. *Eye News*, April/May: 26–31.

Waller, D., Renwick, A. and Hillier, K. (2005). *Medical Pharmacology and Therapeutics*, 2nd edn. London: Elsevier.

Chapter 7
Ophthalmic pain

General principles

'Eye pain makes you feel like hell and look like Jack Nicholson but it's not something other people consider disabling' (Eye Pain Page http://members.tripod.com/lepton/pain.htm). Eye pain is a useful indicator that something is potentially seriously wrong, and prompts patients to seek urgent help. The type of pain varies in terms of the disease or injury and is notoriously difficult to treat effectively. It is important for the practitioner to have some knowledge of the types of ophthalmic pain, to inform patients regarding what to expect, how long it is likely to last and how to deal with it. As a general rule, if pain persists or fails to significantly improve within the expected time period, the patient should be advised to seek a further consultation.

Illness, and particularly time off work, is increasingly poorly accepted within our busy society. Treatments for eye conditions take time to work. A significant factor in eye pain control for adults and children is rest and general relaxation, warmth and a shady environment, and this should be strongly promoted by the practitioner in addition to pharmaceutical interventions.

Severe aches

Severe aches

Acute glaucoma

Effective treatment of this eye condition needs to be given promptly, and will be the major factor in improving the pain. A diagnosis of acute glaucoma in an ED department requires urgent IV acetazolamide (Diamox) to reduce the intra-ocular pressure, which usually produces an effect within 30 to 60 minutes. If this medication is effective, it will have a similarly rapid effect on the patient's pain, further reinforced by local medication to the eye, and so a significant reduction of pain within 30 to 45 minutes is a clear indication of the condition responding to treatment.

Remember that nausea, particularly with acute glaucoma, needs to be addressed concurrently with the administration of oral or IV analgesia. In the event of the pain requiring a controlled drug, bear in mind that a side effect of pethidine, heroin and morphine is pupil miosis which is the short-term aim of acute glaucoma treatment. These controlled drugs should be given with an anti-emetic drug.

Acute uveitis

Pain, particularly photophobia, is a predominant feature of this condition, but patients suffering repeat attacks may have less pain on presentation. Considerable relief is experienced once the pupil is effectively dilated, and once local steroids are commenced, the pain should decline further. Patients report that warm compresses are comforting, and generally wear dark glasses to alleviate some of the photophobia. Oral NSAIDS are a logical analgesic approach to pain control in this inflammatory condition. In the event of being presented with a patient with uncontrolled pain, a diclofenac suppository, rest and warm compresses is advised.

Stabbing pain

Herpes zoster ophthalmicus

Stabbing pain

Patients report the characteristics of this pain with adjectives such as sharp, throbbing, burning, shooting and stabbing, and it may persist for many months. The affected skin becomes acutely sensitive to the slightest touch – a condition called allodynia. Prompt drug treatment with oral aciclovir limits the severity of the attack and reduces the incidence of post-herpetic pain. Treatment with amitriptyline or nortriptyline helps some patients, as does one to two weeks on a low dose of prednisolone. Oral codeine preparations are helpful analgesics for nerve pain but are not recommended for long-term use.

A topical preparation containing capsaicin 0.075% is licensed for use in post-herpetic neuralgia (BNF 2014). It is described as a rubefacient – that is to say it causes a counter-irritation. It is not recommended for use on inflamed or broken skin, but the Pain Relief Foundation states that it can be applied to shingles rash, noting that it stings and burns on contact and sometimes makes the pain worse. This is a very expensive prescription preparation and it should be applied very thinly, and never more than three to four times a day. Cold compresses are a cost-negative, safer but perhaps less effective alternative.

Tyring (2007) suggests the use of Gabapetin or Pregabalin for post-herpetic neuralgia, but these are not appropriate for long-term use as they have many unpleasant side effects. He also suggests Lidocaine patches 5%.

Patients with unresolved pain need to be referred to the Pain Clinic. In the 21st century, many patients expect to be pain and side-effect free. If this is not possible, the Pain Clinic staff will help them to manage their condition, medications and side effects so that they will have the best possible quality of life.

Corneal pain

Corneal damage, particularly to the corneal epithelium, causes extreme pain due to the plentiful nerve supply from the long and short ciliary nerves (branches of the trigeminal nerve). In extreme corneal pain the orbicularis oculi muscles go into spasm, squeezing the eyes shut, a feature particularly noticeable following chemical injury and welding flash. When corneal damage occurs, the ring-shaped ciliary muscle inside the eye goes into spasm, increasing the pain. A study carried out by Lee in 1999 identified that eye movement and light were the two factors most likely to increase pain from corneal damage.

Management of corneal pain is aimed at treating the cause. Never give anaesthetic drops except to examine the eye. If instilled to control corneal pain these eye drops are toxic to the tissues of the cornea. When abused they will cause deep corneal infiltrates, ulceration and even perforation, and are thus only used for examination of the eye and to facilitate specific treatments. They are never prescribed for home use. In situations such as corneal abrasion the pain will not subside until the cornea begins to heal. Many patients benefit from Voltarol eye drops four to six hourly and ketorolac trometamol (Acular) has also been used with some success. NSAIDs used topically (Voltarol, ketorolac trometamol and flurbiprofen sodium) do not appear to delay healing and no adverse effects have been found where the cornea is compromised further (Marsden 2006).

Dilating the pupil with cyclopentolate 1% will reduce the ciliary spasm and give some pain relief. Padding the eye may also make it more comfortable. Patients are advised to take their usual analgesia such as paracetamol and ibuprofen, unless contraindicated, but to take it regularly until the pain subsides. Lee (1999) identified that although 46% of patients assessed their pain as being high on a scale of 0 to 10, only 23% took any form of analgesia.

Children and eye pain

Children and eye pain

In children, pain may be ignored as it may not be not recognised, and it is therefore under-treated. Look for distressed facial expressions, body movements suggesting pain, unusually 'bad' behaviour, photophobia and crying. Pain measurement using a children's pain chart is essential. Fear in the child results in less effective coping on the part of the child, and makes them more sensitive to pain. In addition to paediatric pain relief, you can think about providing a shady environment or possibly a shady hat to help with photophobia. Give extra cuddles, make sure that the favourite soft toy is available and provide undemanding activities. Warmth and the opportunity for additional sleep is helpful.

Ophthalmic sensation table

This table is intended as a guide to pain as a diagnostic feature, and is not exclusive as patients feel and describe pain differently.

SENSATION	POSSIBLE CAUSE
Itching	*Allergy, blepharitis*
Gritty	*Dry eyes, conjunctivitis*
Irritating, sore	*Conjunctivitis, chalazion, trichiasis, foreign body*
Aching	*Iritis, episcleritis, chalazion*
Sharp stabbing pain	*Corneal abrasion*

Eye Emergencies: The practitioner's guide

Dull throb	*Iritis*
Dull throb that wakes at night	*Scleritis*
Pain over brow and in eye	*Raised intra-ocular pressure, acute glaucoma*
Foreign body sensation	*Foreign body or conjunctivitis*
Headache with ocular signs	*Iritis, raised intra-ocular pressure, scleritis*
Headache with no ocular signs	*Sinusitis, migraine*

References

British National Formulary (2014). London: BMJ Publishing Group. www.medicinescomplete.com

Lee, A. (1999). Assessing ophthalmic pain using the verbal rating scale. *Ophthalmic Nursing*, 2(4): 8–12.

Marsden, J. (2006). *Ophthalmic Care*. Chichester: Whurr.

Tyring, S. (2007). Management of Herpes Zoster and post herpetic neuralgia. *Journal of the American Academy of Dermatology*, 57(6), Supplement, S136-S142.

Chapter 8
Concluding notes

Changing
ophthalmic
ED provision

The changing face of ophthalmic ED provision

In order to make efficient use of scant resources, and streamline services, changes are sometimes necessary. Many eye units have re-structured their traditional 'walk in' departments in order to improve their services provision to patients and accommodate the changes to the working hours of junior medical staff. Manchester Eye Hospital was a forerunner in developing an Emergency Eye Clinic (EEC) managed by nurses in tandem with an Acute Referral Clinic (ARC) to which patients could be referred to see an ophthalmologist.

The eye patient management system described below was inspired by the Manchester and Oxford examples and adjusted to meet local needs. As a result, the hospital system described no longer provides a facility for eye patients to 'walk in' and be seen on an ad hoc basis 24 hours a day.

Telephone
triage

Telephone triage

The example record at the end of this chapter can be adapted for local purposes. The illustration provided assumes that a qualified, experienced ophthalmic nurse is giving the telephone advice. General details are recorded electronically, including the patient's own telephone number. This is in case the call is interrupted, or the nurse needs to ask advice of a more experienced colleague or ophthalmologist.

The department it was designed for runs an ophthalmic Acute Referral Clinic (ARC) and emergency patients and their primary practitioners are encouraged to ring the department for advice regarding their condition. If patients are advised to attend the department they are given an appointment time (unless they are acute emergencies).

Eye Emergencies: The practitioner's guide

You will note that the ophthalmic triage nurse will refer some patients to their primary physician. The Patient Assessment – Eye Accident and Emergency flow chart (page 163) gives examples of patients who would be expected to seek primary physician treatment in the first instance. Patients with, for example, gradual deterioration of vision for some time without other symptoms would be advised to see an optometrist. In addition to this a Triage Tool was devised to aid the decision-making process, based on a signs and symptoms approach and adapted from a model used at Epsom and St Heliers Trust (Ring and Linnell 2008).

Some patients require nursing advice about, for example, dry eyes. They might be advised to increase or change the type of eye drops they have been using. A busy patient with slightly itchy eyes in spring might be advised to speak to the local pharmacist. Patients ring for a whole range of other worries about their eyes, for example to ask whether their outpatient department appointment can be brought forward as they have new symptoms. An experienced telephone triage nurse can ensure that each telephone caller is given help and information to suit their needs.

If a patient is given an appointment to attend the eye department this will be for one of the following:

ARC – Acute Referral Clinic

The patient will see a junior ophthalmologist. In order to use the patient's and the department's time efficiently, the ophthalmologist may ask the nurses to do some tests prior to the consultation, e.g. RAPD check, Intra-ocular pressure measurement and the instillation of dilating eye drops.

ARC F/U

An advanced nurse practitioner sees patients the ophthalmologist has designated for 'follow-up' and some primary conditions within the scope of her higher responsibility.

NLC – Nurse Led Clinic

Experienced ophthalmic nurses, who have achieved a documented departmental assessment for competency in managing ophthalmic patients, examine, diagnose, treat and discharge patients with a range of common eye conditions, guided by local protocols.

OPD – Outpatient Department

If an outpatient is having problems that are not immediately urgent, a note will be made of this on the telephone triage form and passed promptly to the consultant's medical secretary who will obtain the case notes and ask the consultant for advice. This may mean making or bringing forward an outpatient appointment.

ED stat may indicate that a patient with general problems, for example head injuries, should attend general ED immediately. Patients with very urgent eye conditions, for example sudden loss of vision or sudden severe eye pain, are always asked to attend the eye department immediately if it happens in the day time. (See the Patient Assessment – Eye Accident and Emergency flow chart on page 163.)

At night

Very few eye departments are able to provide an all night service. The flow chart offers some guidance for the urgency of patients presenting when the eye department is closed. Acute ophthalmic emergencies would be seen in the main ED (emergency department) during the night. Doctors and nursing staff working in main ED are provided with training and guidance as to 'red flag' ophthalmic cases.

'Walk in' patients

Understandably, the general public are not always aware that a hospital system has changed. All patients who 'walk in', unless a clear emergency (for example a serious chemical injury), are treated in the same way as those who telephone. The documentation is very similar. Additionally, these patients may have their visual acuity recorded and an experienced nurse would look in their eyes with a pen torch. The nurse will then advise the patient regarding the need for self-care, primary physician or community pharmacist or book them in for an appointment as above. If the condition is not likely to deteriorate and all the appointment slots for the day are filled, the patient may be given an appointment on the following day.

Instructions for all eye emergency patients on discharge

Discharge

Mistakes can be made and eye conditions can deteriorate. It is important to safeguard the patient and protect your professional position by using and documenting the following steps.

Eye Emergencies: The practitioner's guide

Tell the patient when they can expect their eye to feel better.

For example, the patient needs to know that, depending on its severity, a subconjunctival haemorrhage can take about two weeks to clear. Similarly, a patient with a corneal abrasion or conjunctivitis needs to be given clear advice as to when they can be expected to feel better, for example, 'this is going to feel quite sore initially but should be feeling substantially better by tomorrow lunchtime'.

Tell the patient about their vision.

If you have, for example, dilated the pupil, explain that it will look larger than the other and near vision will be affected, as will accommodation to light. Say when this is likely to return to normal.

Ask the patient to ring back for advice.

Ask the patient to ring back for advice if:

- the eye symptoms are not improving within the expected time frame
- vision deteriorates
- unexpected photophobia or pain develop
- a discharge from the eye develops or does not improve.

Record your advice.

After you have advised the patient, if you have not formally arranged to see them again, mark your documentation 'see (or phone) SOS 1/7 or 2/7' or whatever you have indicated to the patient is an appropriate time interval for the expected improvement.

Practitioner responsibilities

Practitioners are accountable for their own clinical decisions. It is easier to write about and provide illustrations of clear-cut conditions than to be placed in a decision-making situation where the signs and symptoms are perplexing. This book can only act as a guide. When in doubt regarding the need for referral, always seek advice. Carefully document an accurate patient history and examination to ensure a concise record of the patient episode should future treatment be required, or if records should be necessary for any medico-legal enquiries. Use every opportunity for supervised clinical practice and to follow up cases to develop your personal expertise in managing eye emergencies.

Concluding notes

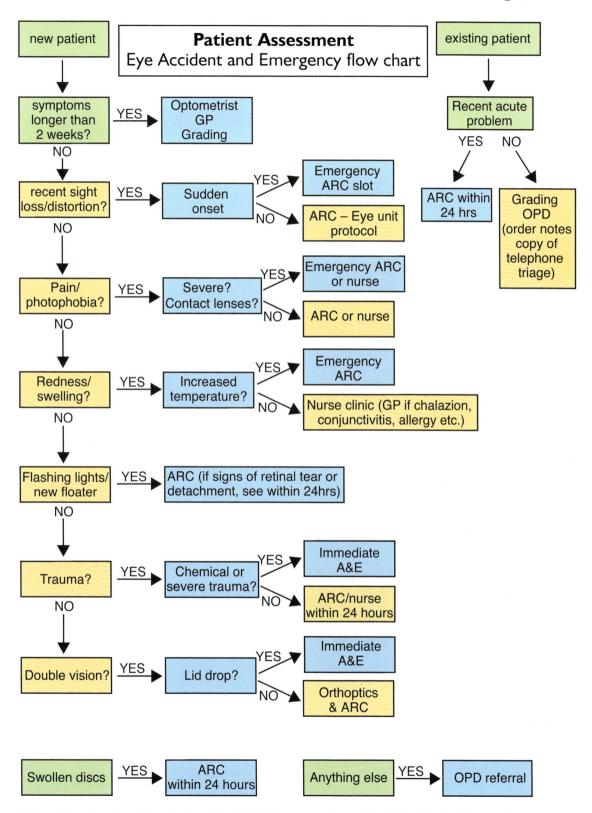

Patient Assessment
Eye Accident and Emergency flow chart

new patient

symptoms longer than 2 weeks? — YES → Optometrist GP Grading

NO

recent sight loss/distortion? — YES → Sudden onset — YES → Emergency ARC slot
Sudden onset — NO → ARC – Eye unit protocol

NO

Pain/photophobia? — YES → Severe? Contact lenses? — YES → Emergency ARC or nurse
Severe? Contact lenses? — NO → ARC or nurse

NO

Redness/swelling? — YES → Increased temperature? — YES → Emergency ARC
Increased temperature? — NO → Nurse clinic (GP if chalazion, conjunctivitis, allergy etc.)

NO

Flashing lights/new floater — YES → ARC (if signs of retinal tear or detachment, see within 24hrs)

NO

Trauma? — YES → Chemical or severe trauma? — YES → Immediate A&E
Chemical or severe trauma? — NO → ARC/nurse within 24 hours

NO

Double vision? — YES → Lid drop? — YES → Immediate A&E
Lid drop? — NO → Orthoptics & ARC

Swollen discs — YES → ARC within 24 hours

Anything else — YES → OPD referral

existing patient

Recent acute problem
YES — NO
ARC within 24 hrs — Grading OPD (order notes copy of telephone triage)

Original chart by Miss C. Marsh, Consultant Ophthalmologist, adapted for this book by kind permission.

163

Eye Emergencies: The practitioner's guide

	Same session	Same day	Within 24 hours	Within 3 days	Nurse led clinic	Not appropriate (see optician/GP or grade to clinic)
TRAUMA	• Chemical injury (alkaline) • Penetrating injury	• Lid laceration • Blunt trauma	• Blunt trauma > 1/52 <2/52		• Corneal abrasions • Corneal FB	
VISION	• Sudden complete loss of vision <6 hours	• Sudden loss of vis on <12 hours (resolved/unresolved) • New flashing lights/floaters with previous history or risk factors (myopia, previous tear or RD, family hx) • Post-op <2/52 – loss of vision	• Sudden loss of vision >12 hours but <1week (resolved/unresolved) • Increased floaters • Diplopia (new, sudden or worse) with orthoptists if binocular • Post-op <2/52 blurred vision	• Sudden change in vision <2 weeks • Single floater with no flashing lights <2 weeks • flashing lights and floaters <2 weeks	• Mild blurring • Watery	• Visual distortion <1 week – fast track macular clinic • Gradual loss of vision >2 weeks – OO • No sudden change in vision (as above) • Bilateral visual disturbance <2 hours +/- headache – Advice – GP • Mild blurring, watery, GP
EYE PAIN SCALE 1–5	• 4–5 Score • No relief from oral analgesia • With nausea/vomiting	• 3–4 Score • Keeping pt awake at night	• Relief with oral analgesia • Photophobia • Post-op <2/52		• FB sensation <2/52	• Irritation with discharge – see GP or advise lubricants • Gritty – see GP or advise lubricants • FB sensation – no hx of FB – GP
HEADACHE	• 4–5 Score with ocular symptoms	• Painful scalp • Brow pain • Painful temples (all with ocular symptoms)				• Tender temples – NO visual symptoms D/W ARC Dr – referral to medics • NO ocular symptoms – GP or OO
LIDS/FACIAL		• New droopy lid/ptosis • Acute swollen lids (with pyrexia, +/- diplopia, distorted vision) • Pain on ocular movement • III nerve palsy	• Swollen lids (normal vision, apyrexial)		• Puffy lids and red eye <2/52 • Normal vision • Watery <2/52	• Chalazion – Advise steam and see GP • Blepharitis – follow guidelines – self treat or GP. • Allergic (sudden onset) – cold compress
CORNEA/CONJUNCTIVA	• Cloudy • Red + + + (with pain)	• Hazy • Red + +	• Clear cornea • Red around limbus	• Localised redness (not sub-conjunctival haemorrhage)	• Red mild to + • Lost contact lens	• >2/52 – advise • Bacterial conjunctivitis – advice first • Sub-conj haem – GP for BP check

PUPILS	Irregular with ptosis +/- pain new onset of symptoms			• Unequal pupil size no ptosis, no visual loss • No sudden change in vision – OO if OO or GP – Grade
OTHER	• Acutely unwell adult with ocular symptoms, swollen lids, pyrexia – SEE IMMEDIATELY	• Feverish adult • Profuse bleeding post minor-op	• Swollen lids – not unwell, apyrexial	• Any patient with symptoms longer than 2 weeks should be referred to OPD unless agreed by consultant or in the urgent/ same session category.
PAEDIATRIC	• Unwell, pyrexial, swollen lids – D/W Dr in ARC - ?Referral to PED		Walk-in with ?absent red reflex (white pupil in photos)	• Any child > 1 month dependent on symptoms • ?Absent red reflex – GP / refer to OPD
OPTOM REFERRAL		• Hypopyon • Hyphaema • IOP >40mmHg • Papilloedema	• Abnormal pupil with visual symptoms	• IOP up to 40mmHg asymptomatic OPD referral • IOP 30–40 - with symptoms urgent OPD referral • Unequal pupil size No ptosis, No visual loss • Gradual loss of vision > 2 weeks – OO if OO or GP – Grade • No sudden change in vision (as above) • Asymptomatic pt refer to OPD
POST OP	• Painful + + • Loss of vision • Profuse bleeding • SEE ABOVE IMMEDIATELY			Post-op <6/12 refer to consultant sec. >6/12 GP to refer OPD pt drop query – med secs

Signs and Symptoms based Ophthalmic Triage Tool

OO – Optometrist
GP – General Practitioner
FB – foreign body
RD – retinal detachment
hx – history
pt – patient

D/W – discuss with
ARC – Acute Referral Clinic
OPD – Outpatients Department
IOP – Intra ocular pressure
Med secs – medical secretaries
PED – Paediatric ED

Eye Emergencies: The practitioner's guide

Record of Telephone Triage Advice – Eye Unit

NHS

Record of Telephone Triage Advice – Eye Unit

Date:		Time:	
Nurse:		Patient's name:	
GP/Caller:			
Postcode:		DOB:	
Hosp No:		Tel:	

Circumstances/relevant history:

Symptoms

Duration:

	Yes	No
Redness	☐	☐
Discharge	☐	☐
Photophobia	☐	☐
Swelling	☐	☐
Loss of vision	☐	☐
Pain	☐	☐
Irritability	☐	☐
Visual disturbance	☐	☐
Contact lens wearer	☐	☐

Impression:

Advice given:

Dr's instructions:

Given appt./Ref. to:

ARC	☐	ARC F/U	☐
NLC	☐	A&E stat	☐
OPD	☐	Cat Clinic	☐

No appt:

GP	☐
Optometrist	☐
Given information/advice	☐
Pharmacist	☐
Other	☐

Notes needed:	Yes	☐	No	☐

References

Ring, L. and Linnell, A. 2008. Streamlining a specialist A&E service to enhance patient care. *Nursing Times*, 104(26): 29–30.

Chapter 9
Ophthalmic procedures

1. Irrigating an eye

Reasons
- To wash out dust and dirt particles
- To treat acid or alkali burns

There is no definitive method of eye irrigation or list of equipment to use. It is important that it is done quickly. Some improvisation will be necessary in a first aid situation, as immediate irrigation produces significantly better ocular outcomes.

Equipment
- Clean, dry work surface
- Paper towels and paper tissues
- Plastic protection or apron for patient's clothing (if available)
- Small jug or plastic feeding beaker with lid
- Kidney dish
- 500 ml sterile normal saline solution at room temperature (tap water is fine if this is all you have)
- An IV-giving set and normal saline may be used if the irrigation is to be prolonged (if you have these)
- pH paper (if you have this)
- Cotton buds
- Local anaesthetic eye drops, if available
- Morgan Lens (optional)

Method
Waste no time. Check the pH if you are able to do so (see procedure 2). Reassure the patient, instil local anaesthetic drops if available and briefly explain to him what you are going to do, as you get the equipment ready. Protect the patient's clothing with a

plastic apron (if available) and paper towels. Position him comfortably on his back, on a couch or on a chair with his head well supported.

Fill the beaker or jug with sterile sodium chloride. Ask him to turn his head slightly towards the affected side. He should hold the kidney dish closely to his cheek to catch the irrigation fluid.

Hold the lower eye lid down gently, direct the fluid first against the cheek, then inside the bottom eyelid. Direct him to look up, down and sideways whilst the irrigation is continued. Evert the upper eyelid whilst irrigating underneath it.

Dry his eyelids and face prior to the removal of the kidney dish. Remove the plastic apron on completion of the procedure.

Remember

- Don't record visual acuity first when treating a chemical injury. Speed is essential.
- Instil local anaesthetic drops throughout the procedure as necessary, as these are being constantly leached out by the irrigation process.
- Use a Desmarres retractor to double evert the upper eyelid if necessary. If you don't have one, improvise with moistened cotton buds.
- Remove any solid material with a wet cotton bud. You may require a fine pair of forceps such as Mathalone's to remove material that is wedged in the conjunctival surface.
- Fluid should not be directed onto the eye from a distance of greater than about 4 cm, as it will be less easy to control and tends to make the patient flinch more..
- Irrigation must be continued until the pH is back to normal. Expect that severe chemical burns may require slow irrigation for up to an hour, using an IV-giving set, with possibly a Morgan Lens if you have one available.
- It may be possible to move the patient's couch up to the sink, and support his head over the sink for treatment.
- Check and record visual acuity before the patient is seen by a doctor.
- Continue irrigating as necessary.

2. Checking the pH of an eye

The pH of a substance is a measure of its acidity. The tear fluid has a neutral reading of 7.2 to 7.5. Readings which are higher than this indicate that an alkali solution has splashed the eye. Lower readings indicate acidity. Tap water has a pH of 7 and is neutral. Some substances fall into the category of being 'irritants', for example pepper spray, used in the control of violent people. This is in fact 'neutral', and will not damage the eye, but is highly irritant and thus needs to be washed out. Always check and record the pH for every chemical injury if you have the test paper available. This should be done at the time of patient presentation, and at intervals during the irrigation process. Leave a few minutes after terminating irrigation before you test, or you will be testing the irrigation fluid rather than the pH of the eye.

Method

With clean dry hands, tear two strips of the indicator paper from the roll. Tell the patient you are going to use some special blotting paper to measure the chemical in their tears.
Fold about 5 mm over at the end of each strip.

Carefully insert the folded areas of the strips behind the lower lid of each eye, at the temporal sides to avoid corneal damage.

The eyes are likely to be quite dry if the patient has already washed the chemical out. Remove the strips when you have moistened a tiny area to measure.

Immediately check your watch and line the test strips up with the colour chart. Read the result after exactly 30 seconds and record on the notes.

3. Everting an eyelid

Reasons

- You suspect that there is something under the top eyelid.
- The person has a chemical injury and you need to wash thoroughly round the eye.

Eye Emergencies: The practitioner's guide

Equipment
- Cotton buds moistened with sterile saline.
- Use reading spectacles if you have them.
- A good light (you may need a torch).

Method
(There are other ways of approaching this, but this is probably the easiest method when you are learning this skill for the first time.)

Clean your hands.

Do not instill a local anaesthetic.

Seat your patient in a comfortable chair, with her head well supported.

Explain that you are going to look under her top eyelid.

Reassure her that the procedure will not hurt, but may feel rather strange.

Ask her to help you by concentrating on looking down.

Don't start until you are certain that you feel calm and ready, and she feels calm and confident in you.

Stand behind her and tilt her head back until it is resting on your chest.

Ask her to open both eyes and concentrate on looking down all the time with both eyes.

Take a firm hold of the eyelashes of her upper eyelid.

Using your other hand, place one end of your cotton bud behind the cartilage plate of the upper eyelid (see figure 1.1) .

Push down gently on the cotton bud at the same time as you pull gently down on the upper eyelashes and out, away from the eye. Using these movements, gently evert the eyelid, continuing to remind your patient reassuringly to keep on looking down. Keep holding the eyelid everted with your first three fingers until you have finished your procedure.

Examine the conjunctiva lining the upper eyelid. If you suspect that there may be a foreign body under the top eyelid, use your moist cotton bud to gently remove it. If you can't see anything, it is wise to gently wipe the inside of the eyelid anyway.

Let go of the eyelid and ask her to look up. The eyelid will return to its natural position.

When you have successfully removed a subtarsal foreign body, the patient will immediately feel better. This is the reason for not using anaesthetic drops.

4. Checking eye movements

If a person complains of true double vision, check the eye movements. There are nine diagnostic positions of gaze. Three are very simple to check.

Looking directly ahead

Ask your patient to look directly ahead and into the distance. You can try to establish the affected muscle in double vision by asking him to fixate with both eyes on an object – ideally your pen torch held about a metre from his face. Check the corneal reflections, which should be central (unless he has diplopia in the primary eye position). Using a pen torch makes it easier to see whether the corneal reflections are normal.

When the eyes are symmetrically positioned in the straight ahead position, there should normally be no complaint of double vision.

Shine your pen torch at both eyes. You should see your torch beam reflected centrally in both corneas.

Looking up

Ask your patient to look up. Check that both eyes are equally positioned in the up position, and whether there is any complaint of double vision.

Looking down

Ask your patient to look down. Check that both eyes are equally positioned in the down position, and whether there is any complaint of double vision. Record any deviations. The other six (cardinal) positions of gaze are slightly more complex.

Next, using your pen torch, ask him to follow the light, along the main eye positions as illustrated in Figure 9.1 (page 172), keeping his head still, and to state at which points the torch appears double, and whether the images are side by side, or one above the other. If any one muscle is paralysed, the arrow indicates the movement, and thus the muscle which would be most affected. (see Figure 1.5, page 7, for more information about the eye muscles).

Cranial nerves iii, iv and vi
The third cranial nerve, the **oculomotor**, supplies the superior,

Figure 9.1

Diagram shows the cardinal eye positions. If any eye muscle is paralysed, the arrow indicates the movement and muscle affected.

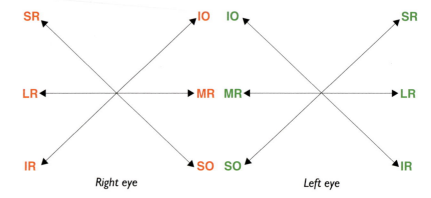

Right eye   Left eye

medial and inferior rectus muscles. It also supplies the levator palpaebrae in the eyelids and the parasympathetic to the ciliary and pupillary constrictor muscles. As far as eye movements are concerned, a problem with this nerve may present a confusing picture, and depending on the severity of the problem the patient may be unable to move the affected eye up, down or inwards. (See 'Visual perception disorders' in Chapter 4.)

Cranial nerve iv, the **trochlear**, supplies the superior oblique.

Cranial nerve vi, the **abducens**, supplies the lateral rectus.

Assessing cranial nerve function competently would be expected of medical staff and qualified nurse practitioners. It can be confusing for nursing staff but usually ophthalmic nurses and emergency care practitioners would be able to detect the presence of binocular diplopia (as a differential from uniocular) and would refer on to the orthoptic department and ophthalmologist.

5. Checking for relative afferent pupillary defect (RAPD)

Checking for RAPD

This is a test for optic nerve disease. In normal lighting conditions, the patient's pupils will appear equal. In the normal eye, when a bright light is shone on one eye, both pupils will constrict. This is called a consensual pupil response.

It is important to check for any RAPD prior to dilating the patient's pupils for examination. Document that you have done this. If there is a gross problem, this is easy to identify, but sometimes the difference between the two eyes is very subtle. Normally the ophthalmologist would like to verify your finding of RAPD prior to the pupil being dilated.

The 'swinging torch test' as this is sometimes called, is used to check the pupillary reflex. Arrange very dim lighting conditions and stand slightly to the side of the patient, so that she is not tempted to focus on you, but make sure that you have a good view of the pupils of both her eyes. Ask the patient to relax her eyes as if she were looking across to the far side of a field. Swing a strong pen torch beam into the unaffected eye for a second or two. You will see the pupil constrict. Without moving the torch beam, observe the affected eye. Because the neural pathways for the unaffected eye are functioning, the brain will pick up this impulse and will send a signal to the affected eye, warning the pupil to contract. You can see this happen.

Swing the torchlight slowly on to the affected eye, dipping the beam below the nose, and then shining it into the affected eye. If the eye problem is with the neural pathway, the damaged pathway will transmit the light less efficiently, the brain will sense less light entering the eye, and the brain will cause both pupils to dilate slightly, to let in more light.

Remember that the resting pupil diameter is smaller in elderly people and the response in terms of maximum dilatation is smaller (Bitsios *et al*. 1996), so elderly people are particularly difficult to examine.

6. Visual fields by confrontation

Visual fields by confrontation

Patients are often not aware of quite large losses of visual field, as the loss is either compensated for by vision from the other eye or the brain 'fills in' the defect with appropriate colours and textures, so the patient may perceive his vision as being merely 'fuzzy' in the defect area.

This is a quick test to check for a gross visual field defect that doesn't require any specialist equipment. The test assumes that your own visual fields are normal, as your patient's visual field is checked against your own.

Method

Ask the patient to remove his spectacles if worn. Sit about one metre away from him. You should be sitting on the same level, with your eyes and noses lined up.

Ask the patient to cover his left eye, with the palm of his hand, and you cover your right eye, so that the shapes of your visual fields will correspond. Each of you fixate on the centre of the other person's eye.

You test the four quadrants of the visual field by holding up the end of your pen within the four quadrants. Bring the pen tip slowly into your own field of vision, and ask the patient to say when he can see the pen tip. Remember to test within the quadrant, so don't bring your fingers in horizontally or vertically. When you have finished testing the patient's right eye, continue the procedure in reverse to test the left eye. Record your findings.

7. Seidel's test to detect a wound leak

Seidel's test

This test is sometimes used following trauma, for example an injury to the eye where penetration is a possibility, and sometimes after intra-ocular surgery if a wound leak is suspected.

Equipment
- Slit lamp
- Fluorescein minim (a Fluoret will not give sufficient, well-directed volume of fluorescein)

Method

Explain to the patient what you are going to do. Ensure they are seated comfortably at the slit lamp.

Apply the liquid fluorescein directly and liberally superior to the site of the suspected leak whilst observing the site with the slit lamp (using the blue light). If there is a leak, the fluorescein dye will be diluted by leaking aqueous and appear as a green diluted stream within the concentrated dye.

This test needs to be carried out in the context of a full ophthalmic history and examination, as a negative test does not necessarily mean that all is well. A foreign body could have entered the eye at speed, causing a leak which rapidly healed, or, following the original injury, other eye tissue, for example the iris, may be drawn into the wound, effectively plugging it.

If the test is positive, inform the ophthalmologist urgently. If not, record on the patient's notes that the test was done, and proved negative.

This test should only be carried out by competent ophthalmic experienced personnel.

8. Corneal staining with fluorescein

Corneal staining

Remember:

- When you are going to use fluorescein, always make sure that the patient has first removed any contact lenses. This is because contact lenses readily absorb and retain fluorescein and could be ruined.
- Fluorescein provides an ideal growing medium for pseudomonas infections and minims contain no preservative and so should be used carefully with this in mind.
  They are not multi-use.
- Don't use fluorescein prior to taking swabs for chlamydia. In testing conjunctival swabs, the infected cells are stained with a fluorescein labelled monoclonal antibody (Holland *et al.* 2006). Therefore, if you suspect chlamydial infection, do not instil fluorescein until after you have taken swabs for culture, as this will compromise an entire automated batch of swabs from many other patients.
- Use fluorescein sparingly, after you have fully assessed the anterior parts of the eye, as it will be temporarily absorbed into the aqueous and vitreous and may affect subsequent examinations and treatments.
- Fluorescein is water soluble, and accidental spillage onto clothing will wash out using a normal washing machine cycle.

Method

When using minims, ask the patient to look up, pull the lower eyelid gently down and away from the eye, and squeeze a single drop into the pocket between the lower eyelid and the eye (known as the lower fornix).

Fluorets are paper strips impregnated with fluorescein and can only be used for single patients. Peel the tiny envelope open, and carefully remove the Fluoret, without touching the orange area, which is impregnated with fluorescein. Use a drop from a minim of normal saline to carefully wet the fluorescein dye. Gently touch this into the lower fornix. If you are experienced, one Fluoret is sufficient to stain both eyes (consider cross-infection first). Be very careful with Fluorets, as accidentally releasing the drop from the end of a Fluoret onto the patient's clothing is easy to do.

Examination

Ask the patient not to squeeze their eyes shut when drops are instilled but to blink gently to allow the fluorescein to spread across the surface of the eye. Fluorescein stains green, indicating epithelial loss on the cornea and conjunctiva from, for example, abrasions or chemical injuries.

Arrange very dull lighting conditions. Check for corneal and conjunctival staining using a slit lamp or a torch with a cobalt blue filter attached and the naked eye or a magnifying glass.

Abnormal tear break up time (TBUT) is the most popular test for the diagnosis of dry eye. It is assessed by instilling a drop of fluorescein and observing the tear meniscus through the slit lamp, using the cobalt blue filter. The normal tear film, as stained by fluorescein, begins to break up after about 10 to 12 seconds. Dry patches develop and the patient has an urge to blink. A tear film break up time of less than ten seconds is considered to indicate a dry eye (Kaiser *et al.* 2004).

9. Application of heat to the eyelids

Applying heat to the eyelids

In the past, application of heat to the eyelids and all the claims associated with it were unsubstantiated by published research but are held by many ophthalmic practitioners to be justified by practical experience and observation. This was considered to be one of those areas where practice knowledge could be deemed to gain its credibility from 'a paradigm of clinical research focusing on individual therapeutic encounters' (Rolfe 1998).

However, Nadler *et al.* (2004) suggested that moist heat applied to painful areas warms the tissues faster than dry heat, but did not find it to be therapeutically superior to dry heat. They found that a continuous low level of heat was therapeutic in pain control for a variety of painful conditions (but they did not examine eye pain). They stressed that great caution should always be used in the application of heat.

Application of moist heat to the eyelids is thought to be effective in three ways:

- The heat promotes local dilation of blood vessels, increasing the blood circulation to the eyelids and anterior parts of the eye. For patients with anterior uveitis and synechiae (areas where the posterior surface of the iris is stuck to the lens as part of the inflammatory process), the local dilation of blood vessels may increase the uptake of dilating eye drops.
- For eyelid problems such as blocked meibomian glands and styes, steam moistens and loosens secretions in blocked glands (Olson *et al.* 2003).
- Patients report that they find the heat comforting to the acute pain of both eyelid conditions and anterior uveitis.

Method

Use a thermos flask partially filled with boiled water, in a sink or bowl. Ask the patient to close the eyelids on the affected side and lean over the opening of the flask. The patient should do this for 10 to 15 minutes, replenishing the hot water as required and being extremely careful.

Steaming may be used as a single procedure for promoting the absorption of eye drops to dilate the pupil in a clinical situation or twice a day at home to promote the resolution of a cyst or stye. Warm compresses are an alternative to steam treatment for children or vulnerable patients. Use a small clean pad of cotton wool or material soaked in warm water and cover the eyelids for a minute or two and repeat several times. Be extremely careful regarding the temperature of the compresses. 'Hand hot' water for the adult can be too warm for the delicate tissues around a child's eyes.

Ward *et al.* (2006) suggest a novel method of applying warm heat to the eyelids which entails filling a surgical glove with hot water, tying a knot at the wrist and then asking the patient to apply it, perhaps wrapped in a cover to the closed eye. They comment that many patients find this extremely soothing to an inflammatory eye condition.

An eye bag or mask filled with linseed is now available and is microwaved for one minute. This is often preferred by some, as it is less labour intensive.

References

Bitsios, P., Prettyman, R. and Szabadi, E. (1996). Changes in autonomic function with age: A study of papillary kinetics in healthy young and old people. *Age and Ageing*, 25(6): 432–438.

Holland, J., Faal, N., Saar, I., Joof, H., Laye, M., Cameron, E., Pemberton-Piggott, F., Dockrel, H., Bailey, R. and Mabey, D. (2006). The frequency of Chlamydial Trachoma major outer membrane Protein specific CD8+ T Lymphocytes in active Trachoma. *Infection and Immunity*, **74**(3): 1565–1572.

Kaiser, P., Friedman, N. and Pineda, R. (2004). *The Massachusetts Eye and Ear Infirmary Manual of Ophthalmology*, 2nd edn. Philadelphia: Saunders.

Nadler, S., Weingand, K. and Kruse, R. (2004). The physiologic basis and clinical applications of cryotherapy and thermotherapy for the pain practitioner. *Pain Physician*, **7**: 395–399.

Olson, M., Korb, D. and Greiner, J. (2003). Increase in tear film lipid layer thickness following treatment with warm compresses in patients with meibomian gland dysfunction. *Eye and Contact Lens Science and Clinical Practice*, 29(2): 96–99.

Rolfe, G. (1998). The theory-practice gap in nursing: from research-based practice to practitioner-based research. *Journal of Advanced Nursing*, **28**(3): 672–679.

Ward, B., Raynel, S. and Catt, G. (2000). The uveal tract, In Marsden, J. (Ed). *Ophthalmic Care*. Chichester: Wiley.

Glossary of ophthalmic terms

Accommodation
The process by which the ciliary muscles inside the eye contract or relax to increase or decrease the refractive power of the eye's natural lens.

Acanthamoeba keratitis
An infection of the cornea by a tiny amoeba, often caused by washing contact lenses in infected water, followed by poor contact lens hygiene.

Afferent pupillary defect
A failure of a nerve pathway from one of the eyes to transmit a message to the brain.

Amaurosis fugax
A sudden, transient loss of vision affecting only one eye.

Amblyopic eye
A normal eye that doesn't see clearly even with spectacles, often caused by inadequately treated squint.

Anaesthetic cornea
Loss of sensation in the cornea, often caused by viral keratitis. The condition is said to be potentially blinding, as it can lead to major infection and trauma to the cornea going undetected.

Anterior chamber
The space between the anterior surface of the iris and the posterior of the cornea.

Anti-VEGF treatment
A group of drugs used to counteract the effect of the vascular endothelial growth factor, reducing new blood vessel growth and oedema.

Astigmatism
An irregular shape to the front of the cornea which, without spectacle correction, may cause a varying degree of visual distortion.

Aqueous humour
The transparent fluid which fills the anterior chamber of the eye.

Bifocal spectacles
Spectacles with clearly defined areas for distant and near vision.

Blepharospasm
A sustained involuntary spasm of the muscles controlling the eyelids, causing them to be squeezed shut.

Blow out fracture
A fracture of the orbital floor, causing some of the orbital contents to prolapse into the maxillary sinus.

Branch vein occlusion (BRVO)
Occlusion of a branch of the central retinal vein.

Eye Emergencies: The practitioner's guide

Carotid bruit
An abnormal sound heard by stethoscope applied to the carotid artery, indicating partial occlusion of the artery.

Cataract
Opacity of the normally transparent lens.

Central retinal artery occlusion (CRAO)
Occlusion of the central retinal artery.

Central retinal vein occlusion (CRVO)
Occlusion of the central retinal vein.

Chemosis
Swelling of the conjunctiva.

Ciliary flush
A circle of tiny dilated blood vessels around the corneal periphery.

Concretion
Cream-coloured inclusion cysts inside the upper or lower eyelids, filled with keratin and epithelial debris.

C-reactive protein (CRP) test
Measures the concentration of a protein in the blood serum that indicates inflammation.

Cycloplegia
Paralysis of the ciliary muscle, causing the lens to flatten, as for distance vision.

Diabetic retinopathy
Changes in the visible characteristics of the blood vessels of the retina.

Distance glasses
Spectacle lenses for driving, watching TV and so on.

Diplopia
Double vision

Dua's layer
A well-defined, acellular strong layer in pre-Descemet cornea.

Ectropion
A condition where the lower eyelid is 'loose', not maintaining good contact with the eye.

Endophthalmitis
A severe infection affecting the internal structures of the eyeball.

Entropion
A condition where the lower eyelid is 'tight', tending to roll inwards, causing the eyelashes to abrade the cornea.

Enophthalmos
An eye that looks smaller than its fellow, as a result of a fracture to the orbital floor.

Glossary of ophthalmic terms

Flare
Protein in the aqueous fluid as a product of anterior uveitis. It is seen in a narrow slit lamp beam as a result of its light-scattering properties.

Floaters
Debris in the vitreous, described by patients as spots or spiders occurring in the field of vision.

Follicles
Raised, rounded, avascular white or grey structures containing lymphocytes, found in the conjunctiva lining the lower eyelid and the border of the upper tarsal plate, frequently noted in viral and chlamydial infections.

Fornix/fornices
The pouch/pouches under the upper and lower eyelids, caused by the conjunctiva covering the inside of the eyelids folding back on itself to cover the anterior surface of the eye.

Geographic ulcer
An ulcer associated with herpes simplex corneal infection. Misdiagnosis resulting in inappropriate steroid treatment can result in a lesion becoming a geographic corneal ulcer.

Giant cell arteritis
Another name for temporal arteritis.

Glaucoma
An umbrella term for a number of eye conditions that are often, but not invariably, associated with raised intra-ocular pressure.

Hutchinson's sign
This is when the rash in herpes zoster ophthalmicus reaches down the side of the nose to the nasal tip and the patient is more likely to have corneal involvement in the infection process.

Hypermetropia
Long-sightedness, where a person's distant vision is better than their near vision, due to a shorter than average eyeball.

Hyphaema
Blood present in the anterior chamber of the eye.

Hypopyon
A mass of white inflammatory cells in the anterior chamber of the eye.

Intra-ocular pressure (IOP)
The hydrostatic pressure inside the eye.

Keratic precipitates (KPs)
Groups of inflammatory cells adhering to the posterior surface of the cornea.

Keratitis
Inflammation of the cornea.

LASIK
Laser Assisted In Situ Keratomileusis or laser refractive surgery.

Lazy eye

A normal eye which at some stage was misaligned. The brain never received a clear image on this side and visual perception via the optic nerves and brain did not develop as well as it might have done.

LogMAR test chart

A visual acuity testing chart that follows the principle of logarithmic size progression and is considered to be the gold standard for the assessment of distance vision.

Macular oedema

An accumulation of fluid within the retina at the macular area.

Meibomianitis

Inflammation of the meibomian glands in the eyelids.

Micropsia

A perceptual reduction in the size of objects viewed with the affected eye. This indicates serious macular pathology.

Monocular diplopia

Double vision perceived by only one eye.

Myopia

Short sightedness, where a person's near vision is better than their distant vision.

Neovascularisation

The development of abnormal new blood vessels. In the eye this may occur initially at the retina as a result of retinal ischaemia. Unchecked, new vessels may grow forward over the iris and into the drainage angle.

Optic disc

At the back of the eye the sclera is pierced by the optic nerve, central retinal artery and central retinal vein. It appears as a slightly depressed area – the optic disc. It contains no rods or cones, and is therefore the 'blind spot' of the eye.

Ophthalmologist

A qualified doctor who is undertaking further studies in ophthalmology or who already holds post-registration qualifications in this field.

Ophthalmoscope

An instrument for examining the vitreous, retina or optic disc. It may be a 'direct ophthalmoscope', held directly to the examiner's eye or an 'indirect ophthalmoscope' which shines a beam of light from a band on the examiner's head through a magnifying glass into the patient's eye. The indirect ophthalmoscope produces an inverted view of the retina. It is better for examining the retinal periphery.

Optometrist

Previously known as ophthalmic opticians, optometrists are primary healthcare specialists trained to examine the eyes to detect defects in vision, ocular diseases or abnormalities.

Glossary of ophthalmic terms

Orthoptic department
Literally, 'orthoptic' means straight eyes. This department concentrates on diagnosing, treating and advising on disorders of vision and defects of eye movements.

Papillae
These tiny raised structures are filled with vascular cores and are a non-specific sign of conjunctival inflammation or allergy.

Papilloedema
A swollen optic disc with blurred edges and dilated superficial capillaries.

Photokeratitis
The medical term for 'arc eye' or 'welding flash'.

Photopsia
'Flashing lights' perceived in response to an abnormal pull on the retina from shrinking vitreous.

Photophobia
Light sensitivity.

Pingueculum
Small, round, yellowish lumps appearing on the conjunctiva on either side of the cornea in the positions 9 and 3 o'clock. These are the result of conjunctival degeneration and are benign.

Posterior chamber
The aqueous-filled space behind the iris and in front of the lens.

Presbyopia
Loss of accommodation in the lens due to ageing.

Proptosis
Protrusion of one or both eyes.

Pterygium
A superficial, fleshy, vascular wing of conjunctiva which slowly extends onto the cornea, and may eventually cover the pupillary area.

Ptosis
A condition when the affected upper eyelid or eyelids hang in a lower position than normal, which may affect vision.

Reading glasses
Used to correct presbyopia (see above).

Superficial punctate keratitis
SPKs are tiny diffuse corneal lesions, with many varied causes, for example 'dry eye', severe conjunctivitis, ultraviolet light exposure or a chemical splash.

Sympathetic ophthalmitis
This is a bilateral severe uveitis. An inflammation occurs in the 'good' eye (sympathising eye), following a severe injury to the fellow (exciting) eye days, months or even years before. Without treatment, the 'sympathising' eye may go blind.

Trichiasis
Eyelashes which grow unevenly, usually in response to chronic eyelid inflammation.

Varifocal spectacles
These work on a similar principle to bifocals, except that instead of a hard line between the distance and near sections, the lenses slowly merge, providing some correction for the intermediate distance.

Visual obscurations
Episodes of loss of vision lasting just a few seconds that resolve completely.

Index

abdominal pain *50*

acanthamoeba keratitis *99–100*

acetazolamide *51, 61, 143*

aciclovir *89, 99, 113, 146, 154*

acids, injuries caused by *38, 39, 42, 167*

acne rosacea *116*

acute referral clinic *159, 160*

ageing *65*; *see also elderly people*

AIDS *62, 90, 101*

alcohol and glaucoma *49*

alkalis, injuries caused by *38, 39, 40, 167*

allergies *20, 80, 81, 117, 146*

allodynia *154*

amaurosis fugax *59, 60, 64, 67*

amblyopia *8, 23, 24, 81*

amitriptyline *89, 154*

amphetamines *30*

anaesthetics
  general *49*
  local *26, 39, 79, 80, 86–87, 95, 148, 167*

analgesia *52, 83, 91, 128, 154, 156*
  over-the-counter *80, 86, 87, 99, 113*

anatomy of the eye *1–16*

anisocoria *30*

ankylosing spondylitis *101*

anterior chamber *31, 33, 48, 69*
  blood in *70*
  white cells in *97, 102*

antibiotic treatment *4, 41–43, 47, 81, 126, 138*
  bacteriocidal *144, 145*
  bacteriostatic *144, 145*
  eye drops *84, 91, 144, 145*
  intravenous *57, 92*
  ointment *80, 82, 83, 84, 86, 93, 100, 120, 121, 122, 144–145*
  oral *91, 116*
  systemic *54, 91, 116, 120, 122, 129*

anti-emetics *49, 52, 154*

antihistamines *49, 124, 125, 145, 146*

antimuscarinic eye drops *49, 142, 149, 150*

anti-VEGF agents *63*

antivirals *146*

appetite, loss of *67*

apraclonidine *51, 143*

aqueous flare *31–32*

aqueous humour *7, 10, 11, 13, 48, 51, 143*

arc eye *83*

arcus senilis *114, 137*

assessment *163–165*
  initial *17–32*

aspirin *59, 61, 64, 131*

astigmatism *104*

atrial fibrillation *58, 60*

atropine *30, 149, 150*

aura *35*

autoimmune disorders *103, 135*

azithromycin *116*

babies, eye infections in *53–54, 90–91*

bandage contact lens *93*

basal cell carcinomas (BCCs) *117*

Bell's palsy *96, 111–113*

Bimatoprost *29*

binocular magnifier *25*

black eye *77–78*

blepharitis *27, 96, 98, 114, 115, 119, 122*

blepharospasm *42, 43, 83, 92*

blindness *67, 81, 99*

blink reflex *112*

blood clot *71*

blood-clotting disorder *59, 132*

blood tests *59, 63, 67, 68, 105*

'blow out fracture' *1, 46, 76*

bowel disorders *135*

Bowman's membrane *9*

brain tumour *see tumour*

branch retinal artery occlusion (BRAO) *59, 61–62*

branch vein occlusion *52, 63*

canal of Shlemm *11, 12*

canaliculus *78*

capsaicin *154–155*

cardinal eye positions *171, 172*

carmellose sodium *147*

carotid artery disease *34*

cataracts *12, 53, 104, 146, 148*

cellulitis *2, 27, 37, 55, 56, 57, 120, 122*

central retinal artery occlusion (CRAO) *60, 63*

central retinal vein occlusion (CRVO) *52, 62–63*

cephalosporins *57*

cerebral aneurysm *106*

cerebrovascular accident (CVA) *34, 67*

cerebrovascular disease *58*

chalazion *114, 120–121, 144*

checking pH *159*

chemosis *57, 129*

chicken pox *88*

children
   common eye problems *81, 83, 91,*
     114, 123, 126, 127, 150
   eye pain *156*
   local anaesthetics *148*

chlamydia *54, 128, 175*

chloramphenicol *80, 98, 117, 119, 126,*
   144

chlorphenamine *124*

choroid *13–14, 45, 46, 101, 102*

cilia *2*

ciliary body *13, 51, 101*

ciliary flush *96, 102*

ciliary muscle *12, 30, 83, 106, 149*

ciprofloxacin *145*

circulatory problems *60*
   see also atrial fibrillation

compresses *87*
   cold *87, 124, 155*
   warm *91, 116, 120, 121, 154, 177*

computer tomogram (CT) scan *47, 106*

concretions *27, 28, 90, 132–133*

conjunctiva *4–5, 26, 27, 33, 44*
   abrasion *150, 176*
   cyst *124, 130*
   foreign body *84–86*
   laceration *79, 81*
   pigmented lesion *134*
   problems involving *4, 28, 95, 123–134*
   staining *87*
   subconjunctival haemorrhage *28, 45,*
     46, 82, 128, 130–131

conjunctivitis *5, 26, 28, 53, 57, 89, 91*
   allergic *117, 118, 123–125*
   bacterial *27, 55, 120, 126, 127–128, 144*
   chemical *43, 81*
   chlamydial *122, 128, 151*
   differential diagnosis of *33, 129*
   follicular *117*
   hay fever *125–126*
   toxic *117*
   viral *127–128, 131*

contact lenses *4, 10, 28, 70, 93–95*

and infections *93–95, 96, 99*
   'lost' *95*
   and eye medication *142–143*
   overuse *93, 96*
   removing *42, 43, 175*

contraceptive pill *62*

cornea *4, 6, 7, 9, 10, 26, 28, 33, 78, 89,*
   146
   abnormal contour *104*
   abrasion *55, 80, 82, 85, 92, 95, 96,*
     122, 150, 155, 176
   arcus senilis *137*
   erosion *89, 92*
   foreign body *84–86, 96*
   infection *54, 93–97*
   inflammation *90, 93*
   keeping moist *78, 79, 87, 93, 113,*
     147
   neovascularisation *94*
   oedema *48, 50, 87*
   pain *149, 155–156*
   scarring *38, 85*
   staining *41, 71, 80, 87, 92, 97, 175*
   stroma *9, 38, 93*
   ulceration *70, 93–96, 98, 99, 122, 144*
   white area *100*
   wounds *44, 45, 46, 148*

coronary artery disease *62, 137*

'count fingers' *23, 48*

cranial nerves *105, 106, 111, 118, 177*

C-reactive protein test *67*

crepitus *75*

CRP, raised *35*

cryotherapy *66, 122*

CS spray *42*

'curtain' *59, 66*

cyclopentolate *83, 87, 149, 150, 156*

cycloplegia *see pupil dilation*

cycloplegics *83*

cysts *27, 28, 55, 91, 121*

cytomegalovirus (CMV) *103*

dacryocele *91*

dacryocystitis, acute *90–91*

dacryocystorhinostomy *92*

dementia *96*

dermatitis *42*

demodex mites *114, 115*

Descemet's membrane *9*

Desmarres retractor *168*

diabetes *20, 34, 58, 62, 64, 66, 96, 103, 106, 120, 132, 150*

diabetic retinopathy *52*

differential diagnosis of emergency eye conditions *35*

dilator pupillae *12*

diplopia *see double vision*

discharge (from the eye) *27, 33*

diuretics *51*

documentation *20, 23, 35, 40, 89, 153, 154*

double vision *8, 29, 57, 79, 101–103, 104–106, 171*

drainage angle *10–12, 53*

driving and vision *24, 69, 105, 150, 185*

drugs *29, 49, 141–151*
   misuse of *30, 59*
   muscarinic *52*

dry eye disease *115, 176*

dry eyes *41, 96, 98, 111, 112, 114, 122, 123, 131, 137–138*

Dua's layer *10*

ectropion *96, 111, 112*

elderly people, common eye problems in *18, 51, 122*
   arcus senilis *137*
   dry eyes *137*

ectropion *96*

glaucoma *48*

herpes zoster *90*

hyperglycaemia *137*

padding *83*

retinal detachment *65*

temporal arteritis *66*

trichiasis *122*

endophthalmitis *107*

endothelium *10, 93*

enophthalmos *76*

entropion *111, 122*

epilepsy *36, 143*

episcleritis *89, 101, 135, 146, 150*

epithelium *9, 28, 84, 87, 92, 93*

erythema *42*

erythromycin *54*

erythrocyte sedimentation rate (ESR) *35, 59, 63, 67*

eye drops *13, 26, 30, 41, 43, 141–142*

anaesthetic *148, 167, 168*
   and contact lens wear *142*

antimuscarinic *149*

diagnostic *150–151*

and glaucoma *143–144*

mydriatic *49*

parasympatholytics *149*

steroid *96, 98, 99, 102–103, 146–147*

sympathomimetic *149–150*

Voltarol *83, 87, 155, 156*

   see also anaesthetics, local; antibiotic treatment

eye examination *18, 25*

eye make-up *116, 124, 125*

eye massage *61*

eye movements *29, 46, 58, 77, 84, 105, 106, 171–172*

eye muscles *7–8, 54, 105, 171–172*

eye patching *83–84*

eye, structure of *8*

eye washing solutions *7, 40*

eyelashes *3, 27, 115*
   removal *120, 122*

eyelids *2–4, 27, 33, 43, 45, 86, 111, 114, 167*
   clinical significance of *4*
   drooping *106*
   eczema *123*
   everting *3, 39, 40, 54, 80, 95, 121, 168, 169–170*
   heat application *176–178*
   hygiene *116, 127*
   laceration *78–79*
   lumps *117–118, 121*
   muscles *3, 86, 106*
   scarring *96*
   swollen *46, 54, 55, 83, 120, 123, 127*

eyepads *86, 87, 156*

face *27, 111–113*

facial palsy *4, 111–113, 119*

facial shingles *88–90*

fan treatment *42*

FAST *34*

'floaters' *64, 66, 103*

fluorescein *26, 28, 42, 55, 82, 83, 87, 92, 95, 97, 122, 174–176*

fluoroquinolones *94, 97, 144, 145*

focusing *30*

follicles *27*

foreign bodies *43, 174*
   corneal or conjunctival *5, 6, 28,*

84–86, 96, 170
intra-ocular 44, 82
metallic 85
radio opaque 47
removing 79–80, 85–86, 148, 170, 171
subtarsal 79, 171
fornices 4, 91, 175, 176
fornix sweeping 39, 40
fovea 14, 30
Fuchs heterochromic cyclitis 29
full thickness laceration 46, 78
fusidic acid 41, 80, 117, 126, 144

glands 3, 7
glaucoma 5, 62, 101, 103
acute 11, 28, 29, 30, 37, 46, 48, 107, 153–154
causes 48, 49, 150
diagnosis 33
neovascular (rubeotic) 52
open angle 14
steroid-induced 146
thrombotic 52
treatment 50–51, 153–154
'warning' attacks 48
glue in eyes 80–81
glycerin, oral 51
glyceryl trinitrate (GTN) 61
Goldman applanation tonometer 46, 48, 50, 151
gonococcus 53
gonorrhea 126
gout 135
'gritty eyes' 115, 125, 147

haemorrhage 15, 62
petechial 126, 128
retinal 104
retro-bulbar 131
subarachnoid 34, 106
subconjunctival 28, 45, 46, 82, 128, 130–132
vitreous 63, 64–65
haemorrhagic stroke 34
haloes 48, 49
hand movements 23
hallucinogenics 30
hay fever conjunctivitis 115–126
head injury 105

headache 34, 35, 36, 50, 67, 157
migraine 107
severe frontal 48, 49
thunderclap 106
heart disease 59, 60
heat application 102, 116, 166
herpes simplex 98–99, 103, 112, 113, 128, 146
herpes simplex keratitis 33, 55, 95, 96, 98–99
herpes zoster ophthalmicus (HZO) 33, 53, 85, 88–90, 96, 103, 146, 154–155
heterochromia 29
history-taking 18, 45
homatropine 149, 150
home, accidents at 38
hospital discharge 161–162
Hutchinson's sign 89
hyperglycaemia 137
hyperlipidaemia 60, 62, 114
hypertension 20, 34, 58, 60, 62, 66, 106, 131, 150
hyphaema 31, 53, 69–71, 78, 81
hypopyon 31, 33, 69–70, 97, 102
hypromellose 147

immune privilege 11
infections 2, 6, 27, 47, 84, 88–100, 103, 107, 170
and contact lenses 93–94, 96, 99–100
in babies 53–55
in children 55–57, 117
orbital 55–57
pox virus 117
sinus 55
staphylococcal 98, 114, 116, 126
inflammatory bowel disease 19, 101
inflammatory cells 31
injuries 19, 36, 37, 38, 42, 44, 45, 75, 93, 96
blunt 12, 13, 29, 44, 70, 71
chemical 18, 19, 37, 38–43, 168, 169
head 75, 77
major 44, 81
occupational 38, 75, 85, 86, 134, 155
penetrating 12, 27, 37, 44–47, 53, 70, 71, 78, 82–86
sport-related 75, 76

violent *75, 76, 77*
internal eye muscles *12*
intracranial pressure (ICP), raised *36*
intra-ocular foreign bodies *44*
   diagnostic tests for *45*
intra-ocular pressure *11, 13–14, 29*
   causes of *52–53, 71*
     measuring *46–47, 50, 102, 148, 151*
     raised *49, 50, 51, 52, 59, 70, 107, 143*
     reducing *49, 50, 51, 61, 71, 102*
intra-ocular surgery *53*
iridectomy *51*
iris *13, 45, 46, 48, 101, 102, 149*
   anatomy *148*
   circulation *51*
   examining *29, 32, 33*
   discoloured *49*
iritis *30, 70, 71, 99, 143, 147, 149*
irrigation *38–43, 80, 148, 167–168*
ischaemic CVA *34*
itchy eyes *124, 126*

keratic preciptates (KPs) *102*
keratitis *5, 89, 90, 93, 95, 97, 98–99,*
    128
   causes *148*
   diagnosis *33*
   treatment *144, 145, 146*
keratoconjunctivitis *123*
ketorolac *128, 155*

laceration *29*
lacrimal apparatus *5*
lacrimal gland *3, 6*
lacrimal sac *79, 90, 91*
lacrimation *42*
lactation *142*
lanolin allergies *20*
laser iridotomy *51*
laser pointer problems *138*
laser treatment *51, 53, 63, 66, 93*
lateral geniculate nuclei *16*
lattice degeneration *65*
lazy eye *see amblyopia*
lens *12, 30, 32, 45, 48, 149*
   malposition *104*
   swollen *12, 51, 53*
levofloxacin *97*
lice *118*
lid lumps *117–118, 119*

lidocaine *155*
light sensitivity *83*
limbal ischaemia *41*
limbus *5, 9, 12*
lipid *7*
litigation *37, 45*
LogMAR test chart *20, 21, 23*
loss of vision *37, 68, 104*
   painless *57–66, 67*
   partial *62*
   sudden *111*
   with pain *66–69*
lost contact lenses *4, 92*
lubricants *147*
lupus *135*
Lyme disease *112, 113, 118, 119*
lymph glands *129*
lymph nodes *128*
lysozyme *7*

macula *14, 15*
macular degeneration *23*
macular oedema *63, 186*
magnetic resonance imaging (MRI)
   scan *47*
malignancies *103, 121*
Mannitol infusion *51*
marginal corneal ulcer *95*
mast cell stabilisers *123, 125, 145, 146*
meibomianitis *31, 114, 115, 138*
meibomian gland dysfunction (MGD)
   3, 115, 116
meibomian glands *116, 120–121, 177*
melanosis *134*
meningitis *56*
micropsia *64*
migraine *35, 103, 107*
miosis *30, 36, 48, 52*
molluscum contagiosum *117*
Morgan lens *40, 167, 168*
moxifloxacin *97*
mucin *7*
Muller's muscle *3*
multiple sclerosis (MS) *69*
muscles, eye *7, 8, 12, 30*
mydriasis *30, 46, 149*
Mydricaine *103*
myopia *22, 65, 103*

narcotics *30*

nausea 34, 35, 46, 47, 48, 53, 108, 154
neomycin 138
notifiable disease 53
numbness 76, 105, 112
nurse led clinic 160

ofloxacin 97
olopatadine 125, 146
ophthalmia neonatorum 37, 53
ophthalmic sensation 150
ophthalmic triage 17
ophthalmoscope 26, 65
optic chiasma 16
optic nerves 14, 16, 68, 172
optic neuritis 59, 68
optic pathways 15
optic radiations 16
ora serata 14
orbicularis oculi 3, 155
orbit 1, 75–78
orbital cellulitis 2, 27, 37, 55–57
    symptoms of 55–57
orbital infections 55–57
orbital rim fracture 44, 75
orbital septum 55
osmotic diuretics 49
outpatient department 160–161
Oxyal 147
oxybuprocaine 26, 39, 83, 86, 148
Ozurdex 63

pain 20, 33, 103, 153–157
    aching 83, 101, 156
    corneal 155–156
    diagnosing 156–157
    in jaw or tongue 67
    on eye movement 76, 79
    post-surgical 108
    recurrent 92
    severe 136, 153–154
    sudden 48, 49, 53, 86, 87, 96, 99
    stabbing 88, 148, 154–155, 156
paint 43, 81
paintball injury 81
palsy 4, 111–113, 119
    Bell's 96, 111–113
    third nerve (oculomotor) 106
papillae 27, 28
papillary conjunctivitis 94–95
papilloedema 36, 59

paraffin, liquid 43, 79, 80, 81, 147
parasympatholytics 149, 150
pen torch 24, 25, 26, 171, 173
pepper spray 43
perception of light 23
peripheral vision 59
pH level, checking 39, 40, 43, 169
phenylepherine 102, 136, 150
photokeratitis 86–87
photophobia 30, 33, 34, 35, 42, 150,
    154, 156
photoposia 65
physiology of the eye 1–16
pilocarpine hydrochloride 51, 144
pinguecula 127
pinhole occluder 20, 22, 23
polymyalgia rheumatica 68
polyopia 104
posterior chamber 48, 103
post-operative eye problems 107–108
practitioner responsibilities 162
Pregabalin 155
pregnancy 112, 124, 126, 142
propamadine 100
proptosis 57, 105
protection of the eye 1–4
psychological stimuli 30
pterygium 134
ptosis 35, 57, 105
pupil 12, 29–30, 33, 48, 102, 106
    abnormality 44, 45, 46, 49
    constriction 12, 30
    dilation 12, 30, 81, 83, 102, 148–150
    reflexes 30, 46

red eye 5, 28, 33, 41, 146
    differential diagnostic guide 33
'red desaturation' 68
'red reflex' 65
relative afferent pupillary defect
    (RAPD) 31, 46, 60, 63, 66, 68, 76,
    172–173
retina 14, 29, 30, 45, 46
    damage 63, 71
    detachment 14, 15, 65–66
    haemorrhage 104
    surgery 53
    tear 64, 65, 66
retinal artery occlusion 60
retinal ischaemia 52

retinal vein occlusion *62–63*
retinopathy, hypertensive *64*
rhinorrhea *75*
rheumatoid arthritis *96, 135*
Ringer's Lactate solution *40*
Rose Bengal *151*
R.S.V.P. *25*
rubella *103*
rubeosis iridis *29, 52*
running nose *42, 79, 125*
ruptured globe *75, 76, 81*

saline *78, 79, 75, 95, 167*
sarcoidosis *103, 113, 135*
scintillating scotoma *35*
sclera *4, 5, 9, 12–13, 82*
scleral problems *132, 135–136*
scleral wound *45, 46, 132*
scleritis *101, 135, 150*
Seidel's test *46, 83, 151, 174–175*
sepsis *57*
Sheridan Gardiner test *21, 25*
shingles *101*
skin rash *88, 89*
sickle cell disease *59*
side effects, drug *141, 143, 149, 150, 155*
silicone oil *53*
sinuses *2, 56, 76, 77*
Sjogren's syndrome *137*
slit lamp examination *10, 31, 46*
smoking *58, 59*
Snellen chart *21, 24, 25*
sphincter pupillae *12*
spondyloarthropathy *101*
staphylococcal infection *98, 114, 116, 119, 144*
stenosis *59, 90*
steroids *68, 69, 71, 93, 128, 146–147*
  eye drops *96, 98, 99, 102–103, 146*
  systemic *104*
'sticky eyes' (in babies) *54*
stroke *34*
styes *27, 55, 114, 119–120, 177*
subconjunctival haemorrhage *45, 46, 124, 82*
subcutaneous emphysema *76*
surgery, eye *24, 34, 47, 51, 56, 66, 107*
  cataract *65, 104*
  eyelid *4*

filtration *14*
  intra-ocular *11, 53, 107*
  retinal *14, 53*
swinging torch test *163*
sympathomimetic eye drops *149–150*
syneresis *65*
syphilis *101, 106, 135*
Systane Balance *147*

Tafluprost *29*
tarsal plates *3, 39*
tear break up time *138, 176*
tear duct *79*
tear film *3, 4, 6, 7, 10, 41, 42, 115, 116, 138, 176*
tear gas *42*
tear passages *54*
tears *3, 6, 92, 111, 113, 147*
  artificial *79, 93, 113, 117, 123, 124, 128, 134, 138, 147*
  excessive *86*
  insufficient *137, 147*
temporal arteritis *35, 59, 60, 66–68*
temporary blindness *43*
testing vision *20–24*
tetanus *82, 84*
tetracaine *87*
third nerve palsy *103*
ticks *112, 118–119*
trabecular meshwork *11, 48, 63*
transient ischaemic attack (TIA) *34, 59*
travel sickness medication *30*
triage *17–18, 151, 159–160, 163–165*
trichiasis *122*
tricyclics *89*
tropicamide *149*
tuberculosis *135*
tumours *104, 106, 113*
tunnel vision *35*

ulcers *5, 29, 93, 94, 96, 98, 99*
  corneal *144–145*
  marginal *114, 115, 116, 145*
ultrasound *47*
ultra violet light *86, 134*
urgent eye conditions *75–108*
uveal tract *13, 101–104*
uveitis *5, 28, 29, 30, 89, 101–104, 107*
  acute *33, 70, 148, 154*
  anterior *53, 101, 149, 150, 177*
vasculitis *106, 135*

vasculopathy 35
vasodilation 61
vertigo 59
vision
    blurred 49, 67, 68, 88, 95, 103, 106
    distorted 35, 36, 63, 68, 121
    reduced 97, 101
    sudden loss 104
    testing 21–24
visual acuity 21–24, 168
visual disturbance assessment chart
    34–36
visual fields 66, 173–174
visual interpretation by the brain 15
visual perception disorders 68,
    104–106, 172
vitamin A deficiency 137
vitamin C tablets 41
vitreous detachment 64
vitreous gel 103
vitreous haemorrhage 64–65

vitreous 14, 65, 104
Voltarol 83, 87, 155, 156
vomiting 34, 35, 49

warfarin 64, 71, 131
weight loss 67
women, common eye problems in
    Bell's palsy 112
    dry eyes 137
    episcleritis 135
glaucoma 48
optic neuritis 68
orbital injuries 77
temporal arteritis 66
xanthelasma 114

xanthelasma 114
X-ray examination 47, 75, 85

YAG laser 51